DIASTASIS RECTI

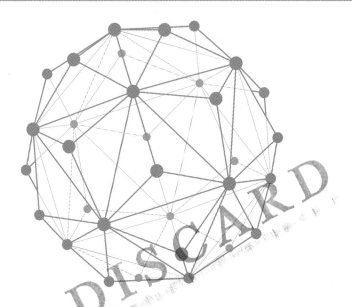

KATY BOWMAN, M.S.

FOREWORD BY DR. CHRISTIANE NORTHRUP

PROPRIOMETRICS
PRESS

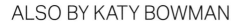

ALSO BY KATY BOWMAN

Don't Just Sit There (Propriometrics Press, 2015)

Whole Body Barefoot (Propriometrics Press, 2015)

Move Your DNA (Propriometrics Press, 2014)

Alignment Matters (Propriometrics Press, 2013)

Every Woman's Guide to Foot Pain Relief (BenBella, 2011)

Printed in the United States of America.

First Printing, 2016
ISBN paperback: 978-0-9896539-6-1
Library of Congress Control Number: 2015953478
Propriometrics Press: propriometricspress.com
Cover and Interior Design: Zsofi Koller, zsofikoller.com
Illustrations: Jillian Nicol

Photography: J. Jurgensen Photography
Cover and interior graphics: shutterstock.com, vectorstock.com

The information in this book should not be used for diagnosis or treatment, or as a substitute for professional medical care. Please consult with your health care provider prior to attempting any treatment on yourself or another individual.

Publisher's Cataloging-In-Publication Data
(Prepared by The Donohue Group, Inc.)

Bowman, Katy.
    Diastasis recti : the whole-body solution to abdominal weakness and separation / Katy Bowman, M.S. ; foreword: by Dr. Christiane Northrup ; illustrations: Jillian Nicol.

    pages : illustrations ; cm

    Includes bibliographical references and index.
    ISBN: 978-0-9896539-6-1 (paperback)

    1. Abdomen--Muscles--Abnormalities--Therapy--Popular works. 2. Abdomen--Mechanical properties--Popular works. 3. Abdominal exercises--Popular works. 4. Human locomotion--Health aspects--Popular works. 5. Exercise therapy--Popular works. I. Northrup, Christiane. II. Nicol, Jillian. III. Title.

RC935.D53 B693 2016
616.7/406   2015953478

For Penelope. Not only couldn't I have written
these books without out you, I wouldn't have written
all these books without you. No, you're not allowed
to edit this dedication. See?

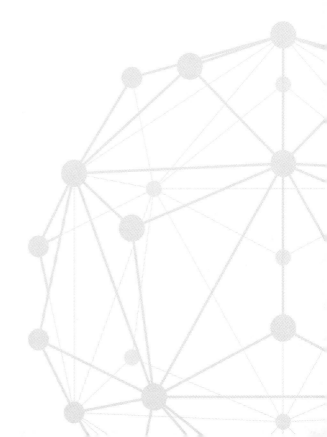

CONTENTS

FOREWORD

As an OB-GYN, I've seen patients with a wide range of issues in the pelvic and abdominal area, many of them musculoskeletal. At best these issues are approached with spot treatments that temporarily "fix" a problem while often creating more long-lasting issues. At worst they're dismissed entirely. And so I've always sought alternative approaches to these conditions—I truly believe that people should have any and all information that allows them to live fully and happily in their own bodies.

I first found Katy Bowman through her revolutionary work on pelvic health. Instead of recommending a single corrective exercise, the Kegel, she was focusing on whole-body movements, including redeveloping the lost practice of squatting, as a solution to pelvic floor disorders. Her science-based work is what drew me in, but I stayed for her approachable and empowering message that each of us has the ability to change our bodies and make them more functional—that you simply "are how you move."

Her approach to diastasis recti is no less revolutionary. This abnormal separation of the abdominal musculature is not, as commonly thought, just an unfortunate side effect of pregnancy. It occurs across body types, genders, and ages. But the prevalence of DR has not been met with abundant research to attempt to understand this issue. Most people with a diastasis recti are told, "Sorry, it's natural, you need surgery."

This approach doesn't resonate with me. We are not passive recipients of diseases and conditions; we are *active participants in our health and vitality.*

Having someone tell you that your frustrating, inconvenient, or painful condition is natural and that surgery or difficult (and barely effective) spot treatments are your only options is both disempowering and possibly untrue. So much of our physical experience is created by how we choose to live—it's not the result of some unavoidable genetic fate. You can learn how a diastasis recti comes about, and how to use your body in a way that allows it to function better, the way it's supposed to.

And you've picked up the right book. In *Diastasis Recti: A Whole-Body Solution to Abdominal Weakness and Separation*, Katy lays out just how we can become active participants in healing and strengthening our core, by changing how we move. From the feet up, and all through our lives, we've been making choices that have created a diastasis recti, whether we've realized it or not. This book will not only teach you the exercises that can give you a more functional core but also help you make choices to keep you strong and vital. Once you realize how practical and how joyfully simple Katy's "you are how you move, so move a different way and you'll feel better" message is, you'll begin to

heal physically. You'll also feel authentically and fully in control
of your body and your path to health. Your mind and body will
be working in tandem to help you strengthen and heal faster
than you imagined possible.

And the best part is, once you start resolving the deeper issues
that created your diastasis in the first place, many other seem-
ingly unrelated problems (we're talking knee pain, backaches,
headaches, even urinary incontinence) can begin to resolve as
well. The practical solutions Katy presents in this book—moving
more mindfully, moving with your community, becoming more
connected with the earth, eating body-healing foods, taking
responsibility for how you feel and how you heal—address
myriad issues. Imagine! All that in a book about diastasis recti!

I invite each and every one of you to take Katy's and my
shared message to heart: You have the power to create the body
and life you deserve. Use it!

Christiane Northrup, M.D.

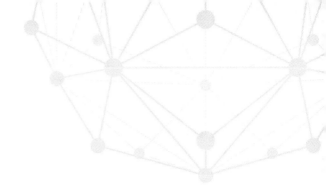

PREFACE

Before we start detailing how a diastasis recti is made, and what you can do about it, I'd like to share my story.

I've given birth to two children, seventeen months apart. After the birth of my son, my first child, I ended up in bed for four days following surgery on one of my pelvic arteries. I was still in the blissful stage following the birth, so the time spent flat on my back (with a catheter, so I wasn't even walking to the bathroom) went by quickly, but when I went to stand up for the first time, I realized that labor and delivery followed by major pelvic surgery and then lying flat on my back for five days had left me without any strength. The hospital staff told me it would take at least ten weeks before I could walk with ease again. The difference between me and other patients, I suppose, was that I knew how to create exercises and a movement program that would build my functional strength back up so that I could stand, walk, and carry my newborn without pain.

I started training the day I got home from the hospital. I

broke the eighth-of-a-mile walk around my block into steps, assessing which muscles my weak body wanted to use with each step and coaxing a different use pattern to get rid of any compensations brought about by my stint on bed rest that wouldn't serve me in the long run. It took me about a month to get back to normal—not to "before the birth" normal, but back on track to where I would have been were I not bed-ridden for those first few days. From there, it was a few more weeks before my pre-pregnancy strength returned. By the time I got pregnant again—a surprisingly short eight months after my first baby—I was stronger than I had been before being pregnant the first time, and my second (home) birth went smoothly.

I'm including this story not for motivational purposes ("I did it, so you can too!"), but because I want you to know that I created and used this program when I could barely walk, with no abdominal strength, following a major pelvic surgery, a blood transfusion, and a vaginal birth. This program comes from my training as a biomechanist and from my experience as someone without a lick of core strength on which to draw. I've experienced firsthand the need to break down exercises into smaller motor skills and postural adjustments, and anyone who follows this program can make improvements to their core strength and separation, regaining the functionality that allows you to move through life with ease, joy, and vitality.

INTRODUCTION

If you've picked up a book with the term "diastasis recti" (DR) in the title, I'm going to assume that you have at least a basic understanding of DR as gathered from magazine articles, blogs, and pamphlets at your doctor's office. At this point you've become aware that the front of your abdomen has split open, although maybe you're not sure how or why.

Maybe you've Googled "diastasis recti" only to find that DR is a natural result of pregnancy—a frustrating explanation if you're a forty-eight-year-old man with a DR. Or maybe you've been told that DR isn't a real problem. (According to one insurance company's medical coverage policy: "Other than its untoward cosmetic appearance, diastasis recti does not lead to any complications that require intervention. Diastasis recti has no clinical significance, does not require treatment and is not considered a true hernia.") No matter what you *do* know, I'll guarantee that some of what you don't know about diastasis recti is covered in this book.

As a biomechanist, I believe that this book is full of information that anyone with a diastasis recti they'd like to correct needs to know. *Diastasis Recti: The Whole Body Solution to Abdominal Weakness and Separation* is not really a book about body parts (though we will cover those in Chapter 1); it's a book about forces. (And before you put it down thinking, "Forces? How boring!" allow me to remind you that *Star Wars* is about a force and that movie is awesome.)

Imagine, for a second, an orange. To break the orange down for the purpose of scientific investigation, I must make a note of each part as I dissect it. For example, the outside of the orange is the epicarp, also known as the rind. The epicarp is made up of an epidermis, hypodermal parenchymatous cells, and oil glands. If you've ever squirted orange oil mist into your face while peeling an orange, then you are acquainted with the oil glands of an orange.

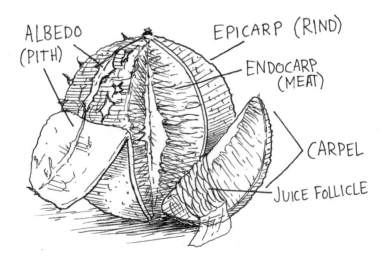

ALBEDO (PITH)

EPICARP (RIND)

ENDOCARP (MEAT)

CARPEL

JUICE FOLLICLE

Connecting the rind to the meat of the orange (and the orange segments to each other) is the pith, or albedo (*alba* meaning white, just like the linea alba, the abdominal structure damaged when you have a DR). Beneath the pith is the endocarp—the part of the orange we eat. Each individually wrapped section of the orange meat is called a carpel. Carpels, in turn, are made up of smaller, individual juice-filled sacs, or juice follicles. Each of these juice follicles is an individual plant cell—a cell that you don't need a microscope to see! (image previous page)

It might appear that I've catalogued all of the essential parts of an orange, having described its appearance in detail, but any good biomechanist will point out that there are parts I didn't include when breaking the orange into pieces.

For example, when you're trying to open a segment of orange—a carpel—to look at the juice follicles, you will see that making a small puncture in the carpel's skin causes the follicles to burst out of the skin. This reveals that the follicles inside an intact carpel are under pressure. The tension created by the carpel skin wasn't visible to me, but it was there. This tensile force is part of the orange, even though it's not visible.

Just as we can itemize the parts of an orange, we can (and many have) itemize human abdominal anatomy. There are the muscles down the front of your belly—your rectus abdominis—and the obliques on each side. There are the abdominals that wrap around from the back, the linea alba down the middle of your abdomen, the guts inside your abdomen, and the fascia and skin that wrap around it all. But just as with an orange, there are many invisible parts—forces—not represented when we approach anatomy in this way. (image next page)

When it comes to a DR, the forces at play are just as, if not

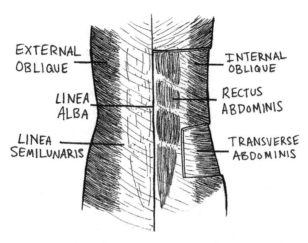

more, important than the parts they are acting upon. If you don't know about the forces, and specifically how you can create forces that pull your abdomen open, then how could you possibly stop creating a DR? Many people, in fact, are actively pursuing corrective exercise to restore their core while simultaneously continuing the very habits that created this abdominal separation in the first place.

This book is about:

- The forces that we create through position, movement, and everyday habits, that make us more susceptible to developing a DR, or, if we already have one, keep us from putting the abdomen back together again.

- How—through sitting, standing, standing in shoes, lying down, getting back up again, squatting, not squatting, breathing, and even how comfortable we feel in our own skin—we can shove our internal body parts up, down, and sideways.

- How sometimes, we shove around the muscles making up the front of the abdominal wall and call it "diastasis recti."
- Corrective exercises, getting *really* strong (although not in a way you're expecting), and enjoying your life more.

And did I mention the forces? There's going to be a lot of force-talk. Just so you know.

Maybe you don't have a DR. Maybe you've lost strength or tone to your midsection, or perhaps you're experiencing other pressure-related issues, like a hernia or prolapsing organs. Whatever your motivation for reading this book, you'll be able to learn about and improve your strength and the way you use your body. Everything I've written here applies to you.

CAN I USE THIS BOOK WHILE PREGNANT?

As I'll explain more on page 13, a DR isn't simply the distancing of your abdominal muscles from each other, but the *unnatural* distancing of your abdominals from each other. And so, the goal is not to get your abdominal muscles sitting side-by-side again, but to restore them to a more natural distance for better uterine, sacral, and lower-back support. You can do this while you're pregnant. In fact, I'd go so far as to say that your body, your baby's body, your pregnancy, and your delivery could benefit greatly from working to restore your functional, biologically necessary core strength *while you're pregnant*. Not all the exercises will be doable while you're pregnant. You might not feel comfortable on your belly or back, for example. Just eliminate those exercises and do the ones you can, as well as adjusting the rest of your movements to the best of your abilities. If you have been given any specialized guidelines (like bed rest), consult with your birthing professionals and ask for their assistance in modifying this program as they see fit.

I HAVE HYPERMOBILITY ISSUES, PELVIC ORGAN PROLAPSE, PELVIC FLOOR DISORDER, HERNIAS... IS THIS BOOK SAFE FOR ME?

Yes. It's not only safe for you—it's *designed* for you. With the exception of genetic disorders, the issues I've listed here are often symptoms stemming from the same problem—a set of forces created by a way of moving over a lifetime. This book is not really about fixing a diastasis recti so much as it is about how to move so that you are strong enough to carry the weight of your own body and not create excessive amounts of pressure. By learning the content of this book and applying it, symptoms of a movement deficit—like a diastasis recti, hypermobility issues, pelvic floor problems, etc.—should decrease. That being said, your ability to execute these exercises safely requires that you pay very close attention to the instructions **(bolded to remind you when form is super-duper important).** As with everyone following this program, I recommend you proceed slowly and mindfully, and enjoy the improvements that you find in your body!

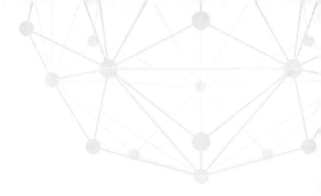

SECTION 1: THINK

THE ANATOMY OF DIASTASIS RECTI

CHAPTER 1

If I begin with a tidy definition of diastasis recti, we'll already be veering off the course to repairing it. You see, DR is a whole-body issue defined by its symptom—the displacement of one or more of your abdominal muscles. Setting up the symptom as "the problem" ignores the bundle of habits and habitats that led to the symptom in the first place. We look for exercises or belts or surgeries to correct this issue that just won't resolve itself because we're entirely unaware of how it was created. Once you know how a DR was created, you can take steps to correct the deeper issues at work.

Imagine you lay beautiful carpet throughout your house, but find that one area constantly fades. You dye that area to match the surrounding carpet, only to find it faded again and again. You head to the store to find the dye, mixing it and applying it to the faded patch regularly throughout the year. Until one day someone points out to you that the faded spot (the symptom) is being created by a beam of light entering your living room

11

(the problem). You put up a sun shade or plant a tree outside the window, and from then on the spot maintains its color all by itself.

Both with the dye and with the sun shade or tree, you alleviated the symptom of the sunspot. But with the dye you were constantly treating the symptom—over and over again. With the sun shade or tree, you identified and corrected the actual problem, and the symptom adjusted to the outcome you wanted.

I'm going to talk a lot about the abdomen in this book, so to keep it a bit more fun to read I'll be using terms other than just *abdomen*. Other terms I'll be using for this area will include *core, torso, trunk, midsection, belly,* and *Esmeralda*. Just kidding on that last one. Maybe.

There isn't a quick fix for a DR or core weakness in general, but there is a solution. By learning the many parts, visible and invisible, that must work together to keep your abdominal muscles functioning optimally, and how to use these parts so they can work together, you can solve the problem so that the symptom you're experiencing—weakness or deformation of your core—will gradually go away.

To improve your DR, you'll need to learn two things: anatomy (the visible parts) and forces (the invisible parts). Don't worry. Even though DR is a whole-body issue, I'm not going to detail your whole-body anatomy (although in Appendix 1 I do recommend a great anatomy reference book. Everyone should have one. A great anatomy reference book, that is; some people no longer have their appendix). But I'm going to give you a rundown of your basic core anatomy, because you need to know more about your Esmeralda muscles than "this is where my six-pack should be."

DIAGNOSIS: DIASTASIS RECTI

Diastasis recti is the *unnatural* distance of the right and/ or left halves of the rectus abdominis from the midline. I emphasize *unnatural* as there is a normal-to-you distance between these muscles that varies based on the natural width of your linea alba, which depends on your particular anthropometric dimensions, age, and gender. In the case of a diastasis, this distance has increased due to a combination of the forces we'll be exploring in Chapter 2, and not usually in a uniform manner (i.e., a diastasis recti is more likely to occur near the belly button than above or below it, and could also be the result of only one half of the rectus abdominis being pulled away from the midline, not both).

A long read of the existing research literature on diastasis recti reveals that there is no consensus on what constitutes a diastasis recti. There is no "normal width" of a linea alba; the anthropometric dimensions (muscle size, body segment lengths and widths) of a person affect the size of their muscular connections for reasons to do with leverage. The DR diagnosis based on an absolute measure of 2.7mm between rectus abdominis halves is more for insurance purposes (you have to pick some point in order to get your treatment covered) than it is for understanding what creates a diastasis recti. You might not have an official diagnosis, but you probably know your body best. And even if you don't have the right numbers to qualify for an official diagnosis, you might be aware that your linea alba has changed—in which case you need to start reading up on the forces that have changed it. In our non-moving population, even those without a diastasis recti can benefit hugely from paying closer attention to their abdominal forces.

THE RECTUS ABDOMINIS

I've seen diastasis recti described as the separation of the rectus abdominis muscle into right and left halves, leading people to believe they've torn their muscle. Don't panic! That's a tremendously incomplete definition. The rectus abdominis has *always* been separated into right and left halves (see illustration below). Although we refer to the rectus abdominis by a single name, it's really a pair of muscles, each living within their own room—their own private fascial sheath—since birth.

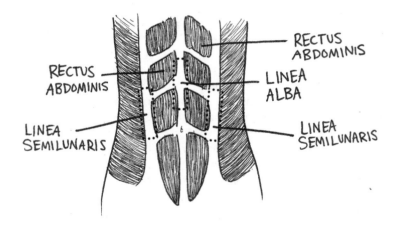

THE LINEA ALBA AND THE LINEAE SEMILUNARIS

Although they may be slightly covered, we all have the three vertical lines that define a six-pack. The lineae semilunaris (there are two of them) sit on the outer edges of your rectus abdominis; between the right and left rectus abdominis is the linea alba. The linea alba (Latin, *linea* for line, *alba* for white) is typically described as a fibrous structure that runs vertically down the midline of the body, roughly from the sternum to the pelvis (anatomical details coming later). The linea alba connects your ribcage to your pelvis, but it doesn't connect *only* to these bones; it connects to all of your abdominal muscles as well.

Unlike body parts like your arms or chest that have bones located throughout, your torso has a large amount of soft tissues, and not a lot of bone. With the exception of the small bones of the spine running through it, the area between your ribs and pelvis is bone-free, and therefore capable of much more movement than other parts of your body.

Being (almost) bone-free in the trunk kind of seems like a bad idea, doesn't it? I mean, your spinal column is there, as are many of your organs, plus a potential fetus or two. Don't these structures warrant the same kind of cage-like protection granted to your heart and lungs? Of course they do! But at the same time, you need to be light enough to move, and bendable enough to forage high and low. Back before food was found in your fridge and potential mates were found online, you had to move. And you had to move to find enough food to support your weight and your daily movement. If your skeleton wrapped around your torso, then yes, your guts-n-stuff would be better protected, but the extra weight of your torso would require you to go gather even more food—a task made more difficult since you wouldn't have the trunk mobility required to hunt or gather foodstuffs. The tradeoff is an abdomen with a system of muscles that function *like a skeleton* when necessary.

If you go into my garage, you'll find a deflated air mattress—totally floppy and, more importantly, foldable. But all I have to do is fill it with air and *voila!*, that same piece of equipment is now rigid and supportive. I don't need my air mattress to be rigid and supportive all of the time; only when I have guests. Most of the time, I just need it to fold up and be out of the way. It's helpful to think of your abdomen this way. Your muscles can become firm and supportive when you need them to, and soft and relaxed when you don't.

APONEUROSIS

In order to work (generate force), a muscle must have something strong to attach its ends to. This is usually bone, though not always. In the case of the abdomen it is the lineae that can have a bone-like function, providing a strong point of attachment and offering resistance to a working muscle—essential for producing force. And like the air mattress, the lineae also fold up when necessary.

Muscle attaches to bones via tendons. But when bones aren't around to attach to (as in the case of many core muscles), the muscle connects to a structure via an *aponeurosis*. An aponeurosis is the same tissue-type as a tendon, but it's a different shape. Instead of being shaped like a tube with a single point of connection, it's flat and has more of a

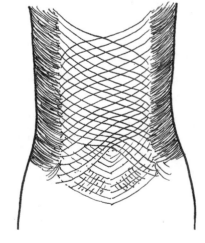

sheet-like connection area.

In anatomy textbooks, non-discrete tissues are isolated and given a name for easier classification as a part. The linea alba and the lineae semilunaris are such parts. But it would be more correct to say that these lineae are areas of a particular tissue-type, created by the basket-weaving effect of all the abdominal muscles' aponeuroses as the muscles move from one side of the abdomen to the other. (image previous page)

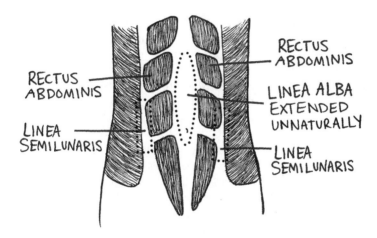

RECTUS ABDOMINIS

RECTUS ABDOMINIS

LINEA SEMILUNARIS

RECTUS ABDOMINIS

LINEA ALBA EXTENDED UNNATURALLY

LINEA SEMILUNARIS

This weaving (the pattern of which varies depending on which part of the abdomen you're looking at) results in a solid structure where every component is key to function.

So, the linea alba is not really an isolated part "where the stomach muscles connect," but a structure created by these muscles coming together.

Instead of calling diastasis recti a separation of muscle, it's perhaps clearer to call it an injury to this basket-weaving of the muscles' aponeuroses, not to the muscles themselves.

ANATOMICAL VARIATION

To keep anatomy lessons straightforward, the anatomical models in modern textbooks and courses are extremely simplified. Imagine the surprise experienced by those who go further into anatomical studies only to find that the textbook image doesn't always line up with real individuals—that many individuals have slightly differently shaped muscles and sometimes "missing" or even "extra" muscles.

Case in point: the pyramidalis muscle. "Missing" in 20 percent of the population, this small muscle sits on top of the rectus abdominis but under the rectus's sheath. This low-force-generating muscle is thought to assist in stabilizing the linea alba, but there haven't been many investigations into the pyramidalis yet, or into how the absence of a pyramidalis might affect core strength overall.

I tend not to think of parts as missing or extra (those are relative terms); rather, I believe that because we are all different shapes and sizes, our parts match the types of leverages we need to function well. Are those without a pyramidalis more likely to develop a DR? Could a pyramidalis occur in those who simply have a particular size and shape that warrants the small bit of extra force produced by this muscle?

If your shape doesn't require that bit of extra leverage, are you really missing it? Or do you have the perfect parts for your anthropometric dimensions?

These are all anatomical questions that can't be answered using our simplified anatomical models. There is so much more to know!

THE LINEA ALBA: CONNECTED TO...EVERYTHING?

Right before I got into this long anatomy lesson, back on page 15, I said that the linea alba connects to all the structures in the midsection. What I mean by this is, the linea alba can be pulled on by the pelvis and ribcage, and by the rectus abdominis as well as by the muscles of the waist. Quick, reach your arms up overhead and grab something off a high shelf or try to touch the ceiling. Can you feel how your (tight) shoulders move the ribcage, which then pulls on your abdomen? I've spent some time labeling your core parts because when you're reading a book about a core problem, you need to know what you're dealing with. But here is what you're really dealing with: almost all motions of the body, even those "outside" the core, *directly tug* on the core. I'm not going to label your arms and legs, hips and shoulders. You know where those are. But what you might not know yet is that the movements of your *entire body* are contributing to the forces pulling your trunk apart. So, let's talk about the forces.

IT'S NOT CLEAR WHAT A DR ACTUALLY IS

There is very little consensus on all things diastasis recti. The visible abdominal protrusions that are the hallmark of a diastasis recti are believed to be the result of a thinned (or separated) linea alba, as I've outlined here. There are other researchers who hypothesize that protrusions are the result of a distortion (stretching) of the entire musculofascial wall, and not just the linea alba. To keep things simple, I'll be describing the loads to the linea alba, but really, what I'm describing applies to any connective tissue (and connective tissue injury) in the midsection.

KEY POINTS:

- Diastasis recti is not a tear in the muscle, but a distancing of a muscle from the linea alba (maybe because of a deformation of the connective tissue sheath that holds the rectus abdominis, or possibly because of a deformation of the linea alba—so far, no one is certain).

- The linea alba is created by the aponeuroses (essentially the tendons) of all of the core muscles, and so each of the core muscles can be contributing to a diastasis recti.

- Your linea alba also connects to your pelvis and ribcage; movements or postures of these body parts can contribute to a diastasis recti.

THE FORCES OF DIASTASIS RECTI

CHAPTER 2

My father was a TV repairman in the 1950s, when televisions were just getting started, and often he'd go out to a house only to find that the problem with a "broken" TV set was that it wasn't plugged in. While electricity might not be included on the "parts of a television" list, it most certainly needs to be on the list of "parts of a *working* television." Electricity is an invisible input that drives the function of the visible parts.

Similarly, you need to be concerned with more than the anatomical parts of your abdomen if you're going to solve the mystery of your DR. We need to be interested in all the components of a working trunk and all the inputs necessary for a strong and intact body. Forces—the pushes and pulls on an object—are essential components when it comes to a functioning machine, yet you will not find forces listed in a human anatomy book. And so I'm going to list and describe some of the forces acting on and being created by your body, that influence the creation or the repair of a diastasis recti. It's really the forces as experienced by the linea alba—the way the linea alba is pushed or pulled—that influence a diastasis.

Even though they go by the same name, your diastasis recti can be different from your neighbor's. Without opening up *your* body surgically, we can't know precisely what's happening in *your* diastasis. Your diastasis could be a thinning in the sheath that contains one rectus abdominal muscle; it could be a thinning of the linea alba in a small area around the belly button. No matter the cause, the fact of the matter is, something had to push or pull on the linea alba for this tissue to break down.

Forces can move your body parts in different directions, like up, down, or forward. You are being affected by and creating all kinds of forces in varying directions all the time. From the traction between your shoes and the ground, to the tension in your calves accelerating your head forward, your movement—and the movement of your parts—is created by the net effect of all the forces acting on or created by your body. What makes a part of your body go up, down, or sideways is always the result of the sum total of all of the forces acting on that area.

EXPLORING THE FORCES ACTING ON THE LINEA ALBA

Picture the linea alba as a long, thin rectangle of taffy running down the front of your abdomen. Below is a list of things that can push or pull on your linea alba, and, over time, change its shape.

- Movements of the ribcage
- Movements of the pelvis
- The oblique muscles (because they're connected to the rectus abdominis sheaths)

- The transverse abdominal muscles, or TrA (because they're connected to the rectus abdominis sheaths)
- The rectus abdominis, or RA
- Intra-abdominal pressures and *stuff* (like babies and intra-abdominal fat)

Movements of the ribcage and pelvis

So: your linea alba taffy attaches to your sternum (which is part of the ribcage) and pelvis. Movement of either of these bony segments of your body creates a particular amount of deformation (called strain) of the linea alba. Different movements deform your taffy in different ways. Stand up and do a slight backbend. Push your hips waaaay out in front of you. Try a spinal twist. Slouch in your chair (really tuck your pelvis under) and then try arching your low back. Pretend you're driving with your arm resting on the center console—or do you prefer resting your arm on the window? Try standing in your signature position. Pelvis twisted? Hip jutting? Chest and ribcage lifting? Can you feel how each movement results in a different amount or direction of strain? Can you imagine how each of those movements deformed your linea alba taffy? Good. Take a rest. You and your taffy are probably tired.

In the MOVE section of this book, you'll be assessing your most frequent rib position (thrusted?) and pelvic position (jutting forward?) and learning some new positions that take the tug off your linea alba, while setting the stage for better force production in your trunk muscles. The ribcage and pelvis connections to your linea alba mean you'll be doing a lot of arm and leg exercises. We've got super tight shoulders and hips, which means using your arms and legs in your everyday life is overloading your linea alba.

AFTER A DR DIAGNOSIS:
TO MOVE OR NOT TO MOVE?

There's a couple of different ways to approach a musculoskeletal issue. On one hand, it's totally natural to think, "OMG, so moving my ribs, pelvis, and abdominal muscles will pull on my linea alba, so therefore I will stop doing any motions with these parts lest my issue get worse." But on the other hand, not moving doesn't fix the issue; all you've done is stopped it from getting worse. And not moving, in the end, results in many more physical health issues than a diastasis recti.

As you'll learn in Chapter 3, diastasis recti is most likely brought about by how you have (and have not) moved up until now. How you have moved has probably been too infrequently (i.e., not moving much more than a bout of exercise, if at all) as well as too repetitively (i.e., you've used your torso for a very narrow range of movements). Consider this: the solution is not to stop moving, but to learn how to create a particular set of forces when you move; to learn how to move in a way that allows some of you to heal and some of you to strengthen. Once you start down this path you will find that your ability to strengthen reinforces your ability to heal, which then reinforces your ability to strengthen, and so on. In this way your body really is a self-winding clock, where striking the correct balance of movement frequency and movement type results in the best outcome for your body.

If you're freaking out about what you have and haven't been doing or should and shouldn't be doing, take a deep breath and know that every step you take from now on will bring you closer to healing.

The obliques and the transverse abdominis

If you look at the orientation of your core muscles' fibers (on page 6), you can easily spot the muscles whose action pulls the right and left rectus abdominis away from the midline. Due to their attachments to the rectus sheaths, when the obliques and the upper part of the transverse abdominis contract, these muscles pull the halves of the rectus abdominis away from each other, deforming the taffy between them. This is one of the reasons very fit and lean people can also have abdominal separation. You can have too much tension in your obliques—do too many abdominal exercises and you'll create a high level of resting tension similar to the tension found in the tight,

MUSCLES MOVE YOU IN DIFFERENT WAYS

Working muscle creates movement as it moves your bony levers—shortening, lengthening, expanding, and narrowing. Muscular motion deforms tendons, bones, and connective tissue as well as all the other tissues surrounding and embedded in a working area. Chronically sedentary muscles that don't work with regularity can also move your parts, but in a less dynamic way: a stiff and unyielding muscle can create a constant pull and deform the weakest link (tissue) in the chain (series of body parts).

A large right-to-left pull on the linea alba can come from the resting tension in muscles that form the sides of your waist. We don't do much with our waist muscles (you'll get a chance to test the tension in your own waist in the MOVE section) and as a result, the obliques can create a constant "spreading" pull on the linea alba that never stops.

A BIRD'S EYE VIEW OF YOUR ABDOMINALS

The locations of some body parts are simple to describe, but for others, it all depends which "part of the part" you are looking at. The transverse abdominis (TrA) provides a good example of a muscle whose location, relative to other body parts, changes as you travel along the length of the muscle. On page 25 I mentioned that the upper TrA can pull the rectus abdominis muscles away from each other. If you look at a different area of the TrA, though, an area below what's called the arcuate line (the location where the basket weaving of the abdominal muscles' aponeuroses changes), the TrA aponeurosis passes *over* the rectus abdominis, instead of deep to (underneath) it.

Here's a bird's eye view of how the rectus abdominis sit relative to all other abdominals, above and below the arcuate line:

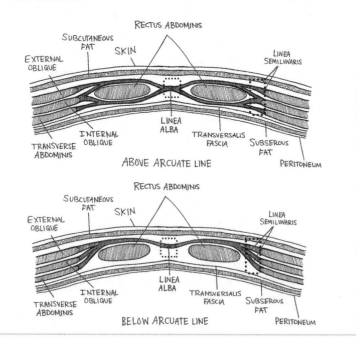

underused obliques of someone who does no abdominal exercises at all. Remember: abdominal separation is not about fitness, it's about forces. The best amount of force is not AS MUCH AS YOU CAN GENERATE, but the amount that allows your body to function optimally.

Intra-abdominal pressures and stuff (like babies and intra-abdominal fat)

It is possible to deform your taffy—linea alba—from the inside of your body, kind of like Sigourney Weaver's stomach is deformed in the scene from *Aliens* where the alien comes bursting out of her. Okay, not exactly like that. Outward pushes from within typically consist of loads that are more evenly distributed, and they rarely involve scales and claws.

DIASTASIS AND PREGNANCY: GETTING OUR TERMS STRAIGHT

If a diastasis recti is a medical diagnosis—a fault in the human structure that is the *unnatural* separation of one or both of the rectus abdominis muscles away from the midline, then it's a misnomer to call a certain amount of separation that comes with pregnancy a "diastasis recti." Clearly, some separation is natural and not a fault in your system. You could have an actual diastasis recti while you were pregnant, but it would be a separation of an *unnatural* distance—the distance beyond the natural widening—whether that extra distance was due to the state of your abdominals going into the pregnancy, the size of the baby, or the combination of pre-existing abdominal fat, baby size, and muscle tension.

LOWER YOUR INTRA-ABDOMINAL FAT FOR BETTER FORCES

I try to avoid talking about body fat because it tends to send people to a place where they can't help but react with bad feelings. Right up front I'd like to say that I do not believe that fat loss needs to be the first step to repairing your abdomen—learning to move better and move more will start decreasing fat throughout your body. At the same time, not dealing with intra-abdominal fat (also called visceral fat) via dietary channels (i.e., continuing to eat in the same way that led to an increase in intra-abdominal fat in the first place) is ignoring one of the forces straining your midsection. If it helps, you can think of dietary changes in this way: you're eating for better forces.

Changing everything at once—how you move, how you eat, and what shoes you wear—is very daunting. And so, I asked a few of my dietician and nutritionist friends and colleagues to supply me with "get started" action items—simple steps toward reducing some of your intra-abdominal pressure by reducing visceral fat. Read through all the tips and see which resonate with you; I've included an expanded list of resources on dietary changes in Appendix 2.

1. *A simple change you can make to lose fat is to drink only water for thirty days. Ditch the soda and diet soda (ditch that forever), the flavored coffees, and even the "healthy" beverages like kombucha and smoothies for thirty days and allow your body to stay hydrated on the original beverage. One exception: if you need a recovery drink, add a tablespoon of lemon juice, a pinch of sea salt, and a dab of honey to your water for electrolyte replenishment. Then, back to pure water! This can go a*

long way in balancing hunger hormones and allowing your body to drop stubborn fat. After thirty days, you may want to continue just like that—or, you may want to start adding back coffee, tea, and other fancied-up water to see how you feel.
—Liz Wolfe, author of Eat The Yolks

2. Dramatically reduce carbohydrates rich in calories but poor in nutrition (bread, pasta, cereals, and other refined grains along with sweeteners and sugars) by replacing them with more nutritious carbs (fruits and vegetables, including potatoes, sweet potatoes, and winter squash).
Here are some simple good carb swaps:
Trade in your breakfast cereal, bagel, or pastry for a couple of whole eggs cooked any way you like and fruit or even some bacon—yes, bacon!
Instead of a sandwich at lunch, pile a salad high with veggies, protein, and a healthy salad dressing based on organic, extra virgin olive oil.
At dinner, trade out a pile of pasta for some grilled fish, chicken, or grass-fed beef alongside more veggies and a sweet potato topped with ghee and cinnamon.
Make noodles out of zucchini and top them with your favorite organic tomato sauce and protein. Finish your day off with some berries and a square or two of dark chocolate (80 percent or higher). That all sounds delicious, right?!
—Diane Sanfilippo, author of NYT Best Sellers The 21-Day Sugar Detox and Practical Paleo

3. Eat at least twenty grams of protein with each meal. That's at least three to four ounces of meat, fish, or poultry, three extra large eggs, or a cup of cottage cheese or Greek yogurt. Aim for twenty to forty grams per meal, depending on your body weight. Protein is very satiating, so it easily displaces more fattening foods, fills you up quickly, and

helps you burn more calories.

It's hard to eat too much protein, and it goes a long way toward burning more fat, faster!
—Roland Denzel and Galina Denzel, authors of *The Real Food Reset*

4. *In order to get started on belly fat loss right away, I recommend incorporating bone broth into one's diet [see Amanda's bone broth recipe on page 208]. Excess belly fat and a puffy, distended abdomen are often a result of leaky gut syndrome. Leaky gut results from stress, poor digestion, lack of adequate hydrochloric acid, antibiotics, sugar, chemicals, poor food, and more. When we have leaky gut, we are in a constant inflammatory state because many of the foods we eat cause an inflammatory reaction. These inflammatory reactions shoot up our cortisol, stimulate our adrenals into overdrive, negatively affect our thyroid, and prevent us from losing weight. What helps to heal the leaky gut is broth made from slowly simmering bones and meat. Broth is full of minerals, gelatin, proline, glycine and glutamine—all nutrients that help to heal and seal the gut lining and reverse leaky gut. In addition, it is simply nourishing and delicious.*
—Amanda Love, *The Barefoot Cook*

5. *EAT YOUR VEGGIES! U.S. Centers for Disease Control and Prevention report that only one out of ten people eat the daily recommended amount of vegetables and fruit, and vegetable intake is really the bigger problem. Vegetables are potent anti-inflammatory food--as-medicine (belly fat is highly inflammatory), and they provide fiber and water to help you feel full for very few calories.*

If you are a stranger to veggies, start small by adding one serving per meal (that's ½ a cup cooked in any manner you like, or 1 cup raw), then build up to six servings a day.

Here are some ideas: Blend up a breakfast smoothie with 2 packed cups of greens like spinach, arugula, kale, ½ a cucumber, ½ a cup of berries in unsweetened almond milk, ½ a cup of Greek yogurt, and you are off to a veggie-led day.

Create omelets with onions, mushrooms, and asparagus, topped with fresh tomato salsa. Create salads that are a mix of greens and roasted vegetables tossed with balsamic vinaigrette for a delicious, complex blend of flavor and textures. Make big batches of vegetable soup that you can freeze and use for future meals.

—Carmina McGee, MS, RDN
Integrative Wellness Coach & Nutritionist

"Things" with the potential to strain your linea alba from inside of you are items introduced into the abdomen, like intra-abdominal fat (the fat that's inside the abdominal cavity as opposed to just beneath the skin), babies, or swallowing a horse. You know those old song lyrics, "I know an old lady who swallowed a horse. She has a diastasis recti, of course"? That song is really about biomechanics and naturally, it's one of my favorites.

When you put more stuff in your abdominal container, it has to expand. More mass in your midsection not only strains your clothes, it strains your abdominal muscles. Like your clothing, muscles can stretch to a certain extent. Eventually, though, they are pushed to the sides, splitting at the weakest point. In your clothing, the weakest points are the seams. In your abdomen, it's the linea alba—connective tissue being a seam between muscles.

But you don't have to have something like fat or a baby pushing

ANISOTROPY

Connective tissue is anisotropic—how it responds to a particular push or pull depends on which direction you pushed or pulled it. This direction-dependent behavior is also found in woven fabrics. Many of the fabrics used for making the clothes in your closet stretch better in one direction than another. If you pull on these items in one direction, you're likely to find that the material stretches and snaps back, but that it doesn't deform as easily in another direction. The give of a tissue is what makes it capable of dealing with changing loads. When you stretch a material "against the grain," you're likely to tear it.

Like your favorite T-shirt, your linea alba (made up of connective tissue) gives more in one direction than others. In cadaver studies of older adults, the linea alba is more compliant (i.e., it stretches better) longitudinally (pulled toward head and toes) than it is transversely (pulled out to the right and left).

DON'T PANIC, there's not going to be a test on the specifics of the anisotropic characteristics of your linea alba; I just want you to start thinking like a biomechanist, looking for WHY a tissue has come apart. Is there too much pull, or is there too much pull *in a particular direction?*

your abdominal muscles apart from the inside—you can do that all on your own, depending on how you tense your muscles. Like the orange in the introduction, your guts are always under pressure. Intra-abdominal pressure (IAP), like your heartbeat, is always there, but not at a consistent level. The amount of IAP varies, depending on what you're doing with your body—your *entire* body. Coughing, laughing, pooping, breathing, birthing, and moving (i.e., your posture and exercise habits) are all things that can change the amount of pressure in your abdomen. Because diastasis recti is a common post-natal injury, it's easy to chalk it up as inevitable damage caused by the ever-expanding (ever-abdominal-splitting) mass of the baby, and to assume that the damage is brought about by a one-time too-great load, rather than by a lifetime of habits or a particular state of tissues. Because men, children, and nulliparous (meaning "not having given birth," a term probably based on the Latin word for "rested"—HA HA) women can develop a diastasis recti, it's clearly not a result of the state of pregnancy, but a matter of forces to which pregnancy *could* contribute.

The linea alba, like the elastic in your socks, is pretty resilient. You can stretch, release, stretch, release, stretch, release. However, also like socks, there is a point at which the stretch is in the wrong direction, too frequent, held too long, or all three. In this case the sock elastic is shot (I call those socks "quitters") and the pair goes into the rag pile. Your linea alba has a threshold of deformation before it gives in to the load and deforms perma-nently.

As I said earlier, all core muscles connect indirectly to the linea alba, which means repetitive motions or chronic tension in any of these muscles—your obliques and transverse abdominals included—can slowly deform the linea alba.

How did your linea alba deform? You might have been standing with your hips thrusting out in front of you, straining your linea alba for the last thirty years. And then you got preg-nant, straining it further. Maybe you've been sitting down at a desk for the last couple of decades and your waist muscles are so tight that they've been pulling on your linea alba for years and years. Maybe you're active, but you've got a pelvis that's just slightly twisted and a ribcage that's slightly shifted to the left. Perhaps you're a tennis player with a crazy serve that's made one side of your abdominals slightly stronger than the other. Maybe you've never exercised in your life and it's the intra-abdominal fat pushing through. Whatever the mechanism of deformation was, it really doesn't matter at this point. What matters now is that there is a way to take unnecessary loads off of the linea alba, a way to get your muscles working to pull the rectus abdominis back toward the midline, and a way of using your body that maintains this core restoration.

KEY POINTS:

- Forces placed on the linea alba deform and damage this tissue.

- Forces placed on the linea alba can be created by:

  - greater-than-natural abdominal contents (a baby or visceral fat)

  - too much tension in the abdominal muscles attaching to the linea alba (the transverse abdominal and oblique muscles)

  - certain positions

  - a combination of any or all of the above

- A new way of moving can instantly change the way you're loading the area of your separation.

UNDER PRESSURE: DR, HERNIAS, AND PELVIC ORGAN PROLAPSE, OH MY

CHAPTER 3

Musculoskeletal issues are typically researched by breaking down your body into parts. Problems with the body are often thought of as either neurological, structural, hormonal, or environmental. A single study will look at the collagen qualities of a group, or their stress level. Perhaps the study looks at their exercise behavior, or their posture, or the strength of a particular motion, or the electrical activity of a certain muscle. Whatever the case, every study is looking at a single, reduced thing to evaluate that thing's contribution to the problem. Scientific investigation, then, is about grabbing all of those reduced parts and pulling them together because, you see, the parts are all connected.

As a biomechanist, I tend to look at problems from a "forces" perspective, and so this chapter will be about pressure and unnaturally high pressure, and its contribution to the movements, strain, and potential damage to your parts.

Pressure is the exertion of force upon a surface by an object or fluid. If you think of the abdomen as two hands (representing your muscle) wrapped around a balloon (representing your guts), then you can see how squeezing your hands (tensing your muscle) increases the pressure inside the balloon.

I also like to think of pressure in terms of how many kids (representing mass) are in a room (representing volume). If you have three kids in a huge room, there's not that much pressure. But if you put twenty kids in that same room, the pressure goes up! Or, take those first three kids and put them into a tiny room; that also increases the pressure.

You can increase the pressure within a cavity of your body—like your abdomen—by increasing the stuff within it (like adding intra-abdominal fat, or a growing fetus) or by decreasing the size (volume) of the cavity through postural changes and muscular contractions. When you add mass or decrease volume, the pressure within a container goes up, which, when it comes to your abdomen, means your guts get displaced outward, backward, upward, downward, or diagonally and start to push on (or into) places they shouldn't.

Intra-abdominal pressure can affect other pressures in the body because pressures in your body do not exist in a vacuum. (Biomechanist joke, sorry.) What I mean is, you're not a floating abdomen. Just above your abdominal "balloon" sits a thoracic "balloon." And below your abdominal "balloon" sits a pelvic "balloon." So instead of the single balloon-abdomen I mentioned above, you can in fact imagine three stacked balloons, representing your three pressure chambers. (see image next page)

Like balloons, the walls of our human pressure chambers are pliable. Muscles and connective tissues easily change lengths;

excessive pressure in an area can easily lead to that area expanding to encroach on the space of the other chambers. If you squeeze the abdominal balloon in the middle, part of it shoots upward and part shoots downward. Imagine how the pressure will change in the sandwiching balloons simply because of something you did to the center balloon.

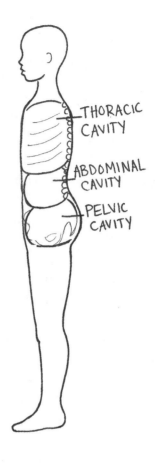

THORACIC CAVITY

ABDOMINAL CAVITY

PELVIC CAVITY

The walls of your containers are mostly muscular, which means you can change the pressures in your various pressure chambers via a series of almost undetectable muscle contractions. Ever clear your ears while in a plane by taking a deep breath and then sealing it off and pushing it around until your ears popped open? You create various pressures all day long—some consciously, some unconsciously, some helpful, some not.

I used to have this horse Penny who was very stubborn and hated to be ridden. Penny used to take a deep breath to puff up her belly so that after I had cinched her saddle around her, she could blow her air out, making her horse waist smaller, knocking me off in the process. She was a genius. You can do this too. Take a deep breath and make your waist larger in circumference. Now, keep the circumference but keep breathing. (Please do not stop breathing for this exercise.) Your breaths won't be as deep, but you'll still be able to both breathe and maintain that expansion. Now try it the other way around. Suck your stomach all the way in and then go about breathing. In both cases you were still breathing (hopefully), but you were able to maintain a larger or a narrower circumference of your abdomen. In each case the qualities and quantities of your breath changed, but you still met both objectives of holding your stomach where you wanted it and breathing.

PLEASE TELL ME YOU'RE STILL BREATHING!

You have many pressure-altering habits and I'll wager that you've been doing them so frequently that you no longer realize you're doing them. I've helped thousands (yes, thousands) of people through the process of strengthening their core muscles, and almost all of them have come to me with the habit of sucking in their stomach. Have you ever wondered where the stuff that used to be on the front of your body has gone? Answer: into your abdominal cavity, just like your cheeks end up inside your mouth when you make fish lips. Only, unlike your mouth (which is fairly spacious), your abdomen is already full to the brim. When you suck your stomach in, the inside goodies (guts) are displaced based on the amount of outside goodies you're trying to hide. Usually, your sucking it in displaces your guts upward, where they're now preventing the movement of your diaphragm. You do that long enough, you just might push them through the diaphragm and into your thoracic cavity,

DIASTASIS RECTI, ABDOMINAL ANEURYSM, AND PELVIC FLOOR ISSUES

Remember back in the intro, where the section swiped from an insurance policy said that diastasis recti poses no real threat to health and is primarily a cosmetic issue? While there is no research proving diastasis recti causes other ailments or vice versa, there is evidence that women with a diastasis recti will have a higher degree of pain in the abdominal and pelvic region (see Parker in the references). In another study, 66 percent of tested patients with a DR had at least one support-related pelvic floor dysfunction diagnosis (you can follow this up with the Spitznagle reference). An association between abdominal aortic aneurysm and DR (as well as inguinal hernias) has also been established (the McPhail and Lehnert references).

These associations are just that—associations—and not statements of a relationship greater than that. However, when you consider how the body is operating as a whole, these associations are important to keep in mind, as they all relate back to pressure. The work you'll be doing for your diastasis is really just work you should be doing for the good of your entire body. The visceral fat you work to reduce, the muscle mass you work to establish, and the functional movement patterns you will develop *help your body* and not only your DR.

The DR is just a symptom—a sign of poor mechanical nutrition. Select a more nutritious movement diet, and your body will be in a much better position to heal DR, pelvic floor issues, hernias, and more.

creating what's called a hiatal hernia.

In fact, the mechanism for a diastasis recti is the same mechanism for a hernia: the pressure on a tissue between muscles is too great, or the tissue is too weak. Either way, the result is the same: a strain to the tissue, in the form of a stretch or a tear. If you were an orange, a tear in your pith would simply leak a little juice, but since you're a human, you leak...wait for it...your innards.

At this point I'll ask you to take stock of your hernia history. Your history of pressure-induced leaks gives you data about yourself, which will come in handy when figuring out which alignment and movement habits you have and which you need. Too much downward pressure (or a weakness in your groin's connective tissue) can spring a leak resulting in a bulge of tissue into your groin (an inguinal hernia) or your hip (a femoral hernia). Too much forward pressure can result in an umbilical (around the belly button) hernia. Upward leaks can push your stomach through your diaphragm (the upper wall of the abdominal cavity and the bottom of the thoracic) into your chest.

Yes, you read that right.

The diagnosis of "inguinal hernia" or "hiatal hernia" (a.k.a. stomach in your chest) is really the naming of a symptom. If we called an inguinal hernia "pressure in the trunk exceeding the strength of the lower abdominal wall," it might seem less nebulous and certainly less spontaneous. If a hiatal hernia were called "your abdominal pressure just shoved your stomach into a cavity in which it does not belong," you might be more inclined to learn about the forces that created the movement in the first place. There isn't a disease that moves your organs from one part of your body to another—but there is a way of using your body that can move your parts into places they shouldn't be.

If you have a diastasis recti, prolapse, or history of hernias, the location of your leak gives you data about the forces you create with regularity. Forces go hand-in-hand with movements—movements we consider exercise and movements we don't consider at all—that create static loads within the torso all day long. Wearing belts and compressive garments, holding your breath, tensing your abdomen all day long, sitting, and standing can all be pressure-changers and thus need to be evaluated as you're trying to resolve your diastasis recti or other core issue.

ALIGNMENT MATTERS

At the beginning of a core restoration, I like to talk about alignment. That is, how your body is organized when you move. Say you commute an hour each way to work, and you do so with your arm resting on the center console. While there is nothing unnatural about sliding your ribcage to the right—your supple waist and many vertebrae easily allow for that sideways motion—the frequency with which you assume this position strains the linea alba in a particular way. So, step one could be stacking your ribs directly over your pelvis when you drive to decrease the unnatural load to the linea alba. What is unnatural about this load is not the position—the sideways ribcage—but the frequency: the sideways ribcage for two hours a day, every day, for, say, twenty years.

To keep things simple at first, we'll strive to find what I'll call a neutral core—keeping your pelvis and ribcage stacked in a way that primes your core muscles for working well—throughout the day. Eventually you'll want to move in many directions and

CLOTHING AND PRESSURE

I can't write a chapter about pressure and not mention the enormous pressures created by much of our clothing. You move through your environment, but remember, your environment can also move you right back. Sometimes the environment is sixty-five-pound--capacity pants encasing an eighty-pound lower body.

Compressive garments can do physical harm, as evidenced by the June 2015 case of an Australian woman sustaining nerve damage from her skinny jeans. Other effects from tight clothing aren't as dramatic, but can be equally harmful.

The thing is, as I keep stating in different ways, you're not a Nerf ball. You don't come with extra space like the foam used to make a Nerf toy. Clothing that compresses your parts comes with consequences, and of course pushing on one part pushes on another and another and another. Compressive garments don't only push on the larger pressure chambers of your thoracic, abdominal, and pelvic cavities—they push on what's inside of these chambers.

Your body is full of tubes—tubes with important jobs. When you push on a tube, the fluid inside of it has to move elsewhere, and the flow through the tube changes.

Here is a list of the tubes that live inside your pants:
• Arteries
• Veins
• Lymphatic tubes
• The digestive tract
• Stomach
• Small intestine
• Large intestine
• Tubes through your reproductive parts

(Clothing and Pressure cont'd)

Here is a list of potentially compressive garments:
- Skinny jeans
- Compressive garments that are advertised as compressive garments
- Tight underwear
- Belts
- Tights
- Tight pants
- Pants that are too small or tight
- Pights

So, anyhow, it seems like kind of an expensive tax to pay for your outfit.

---

assume many positions, but at first, we have to ensure that your movements come from a stable place, where your muscles are able to function optimally and support your movement and not strain the linea alba alone.

For example, stand up without shoes, and back your hips all the way up over your heels until your toes are liftable. Now relax and see if your pelvis floats forward, toward your toes again. Move your hips back again over your heels. The alignment we're after here is one where the legs can support your body instead of the linea alba having to. (If you want to go forward again, do so, this time feeling for that linea alba "taffy" and how jutting your hips places tension on the front of your abdomen.

From the title of this book, I hope it's clear that I consider diastasis recti and hernias to be whole-body issues. Furthermore, I consider diastasis recti and most ailments suffered by most people you know to be *whole-life* issues. Which brings us to the chapter on Nutritious Movement.

CONNECTIVE TISSUE DISORDERS

There are conditions, like Type IV Ehlers-Danlos and Marfan's syndrome, where body tissue is extremely fragile, potentially creating a scenario where normal loads to the linea alba result in tissue damage. The good news is, even in these cases, reducing the loads to the linea alba and strengthening the muscles can result in similar positive effects. Because we, collectively, have some major movement issues and are weak as a culture, it makes it difficult to separate what's a genetically inevitable weakness and what's a cultural one.

If you have a condition that has left your tissues extremely fragile, follow the exercise programs in this book paying very close attention to **the bolded** modifications I've given and work at the most basic level for as long as you feel comfortable. Listen to your body to keep the workload at the best level for you.

KEY POINTS:

- The way you use your body determines the amount of pressures you have throughout your body.

- Other pressure-related ailments can result in similar-to-DR connective tissue failures elsewhere in the body; knowing how pressures are created throughout the body is key to improving these situations.

- It's not only about how or how much you exercise—there's a whole bunch of non-exercise things, like how you breathe, how you hold your body (read: suck in your stomach), and even how you dress, that can place unnatural loads on your linea alba.

DIASTASIS RECTI AND NUTRITIOUS MOVEMENT

CHAPTER 4

Whether because it's difficult to pin down what exactly constitutes a DR, because it's perceived as a natural side effect of pregnancy, or because not many individuals are game to be surgically opened up for research's sake, there's very little research on diastasis recti. There is, however, a ton of research on another connective tissue structure: the anterior cruciate ligament (ACL) of the knee. There are a lot of ACL injuries out there, so there have been a lot of studies into how people with knee issues move—how much they move, what kind of sports they play, how much time they spend on the couch, their gait pattern, their shoe choices, the strength in the muscles of their legs, how they land jumps, how often they jump. And on and on. My point is, there has been enough research into ACL injuries to figure out that the way an ACL-injury sufferer moves is a contributing factor.

While it's accurate to say that in the case of an ACL injury, the load to the ACL was too great for the ACL to bear, a step back reveals that the *leg as a whole* was not suited to the load. Another step back reveals that the *body as a whole*—as a whole bundle of habits—was not suited to the load. In research we try to separate a person from their habits, but in reality, the physical state of your body—the literal distribution of your physical structure—is created by how you have moved over your lifetime.

As I explain quite extensively in my book *Move Your DNA*, there is a large discrepancy between the amount of movement we experience in modern society and the amount of movement humans have been doing for thousands and thousands of years. And it's not only the quantity of movement that's changed; qualities of movement are also much different. Staying mostly indoors our entire lives, we barely move our bodies. Even those who are most fit—in that they get regular strenuous exercise, a couple of hours a day, most days a week—are sedentary and indoors most of the rest of time. If you do a quick Google search on "orcas in captivity," you can find an image that depicts the collapsed dorsal fin (also a connective tissue structure). This collapse is brought about by the limited, unnatural types of movement (round and round and slow and shallow) that happen in the swimming tanks where captive orcas live.

We modern humans barely move, and we have the collapsing structures to show for it. Not only do we need to "get our exercise," but we don't do well structurally when we're sedentary the bulk of the day and thus we also need to move more frequently throughout the day. By this I mean not only spend more time at it, but also move *more of our parts* when we're moving.

If an ACL injury is brought about by a whole body's bundle of habits, we must recognize that a bundle of habits is brought about by a habitat. Your habitat is where your habits are at.

Our modern habitat, for all the wonderful advancements it has allowed, forces us into a particular body geometry. Chairs, heeled shoes, computers, cars—the list goes on—have forced your body to adapt in a way that means when you get up out of your chair to walk around, a great load is placed on your linea alba. Not the muscles of the core, mind you (those muscles are rarely loaded), but the connective tissue that can support you without expending energy. Ever wonder why you like to jut your hip out while you stand? Why you hold your hands behind your back? And why your pelvis rests in a forward position? These positions allow you to stay upright without making your muscles work.

The body's innate tendency to conserve energy comes from a time when food and movement were more organically entwined. When humans spent most of the day moving and expending energy to find barely enough food to cover the caloric cost of finding it, "lazy" standing wasn't a big deal. You weren't going to be standing around doing nothing all that often. But when we move very little, our natural "lazy standing" tendencies are called on more frequently—and it's the frequency of these lazy loads that can cause injury.

Slow, sustained loads in a certain direction (remember anisotropy on page 32?) can deform tissues in a manner from which they cannot recover. Mechanical creep (yes, I said creep) is the tendency of a material to deform slowly under a constant stress. The failure of a tissue in this case is called a creep failure. A disastasis recti or hernia is the result of creep failures. You could also say that these tissues got creeped out. (Or you can leave the biomechanist jokes to me and go about your business.)

The tendency to use our connective tissue to rest not only overloads the connective tissue, it *under*-loads various muscles.

BONE BROTH

"I recommend bone broth to assist in blood building, which is so essential after childbirth. The protein matrix of bone in which minerals deposit is quite collagenous, which makes bone broth ideal. Rich in collagenous glyco-saminoglycans, bone broth helps heal gut inflammation and form healthy connective tissues, including liga-ments and tendons but also the communicative connec-tive tissue matrix throughout the body, including bone. Also rich in glucosamine and hyaluronic acid, in addition to glycine—an amino acid building block—bone broth stimulates fibroblasts to weave the connective tissue web."
—Dr. Eden Fromberg, DO, holistic OB-GYN

There are mechanical nutrients and there are dietary nutrients, and they work together. If someone with osteoporosis supplements their diet with calcium and vitamin D, but doesn't load their bones (creating mechanical nutrients), then the signal to use the dietary minerals is missing and the bone stays the same. And if you're creating oodles of mechanical signals to heal and to strengthen your tissues, but you're lacking certain dietary nutrients, your tissues will also stay the same.

This book contains information on how to create the mechanical signals necessary to restore the core, but in order to fully reap the benefits of the physical loads, you must also consume the dietary building blocks your body uses to execute the "strengthen" signals.

When we order chicken for dinner, we get a grilled breast. When we order beef, we get a steak. It's only over the last fifty years that we've gone from consuming most of an animal—the fat, skin, bones, and organs—to eating only an animal's muscle. If our grandparents could see us now, they would likely be shocked at the waste—of the animals, and of the nutrients.

For centuries the bones of slaughtered animals were not tossed aside—they were revered, for the (anecdotally) powerful healing properties found by drinking broths made by boiling them extensively. Today, researchers are interested in how consuming another animal's connective tissue (i.e., bone broth and its components of amino acids and collagen) affects the health and strength of our connective tissue. Check out Appendix 2; I've included Amanda Love's bone broth recipe as well as the latest research on the health effects of supplementing your diet with these nutrients.

In the end, you are both how you move and what you eat. For the best core-restoring results, you must do both well.

When you've been using your arms almost exclusively for activities (typing, driving, pushing a stroller) where they are positioned out in front of you, your shoulders lose some of their range of motion. In those few times a day when you do use your arms overhead—that rare tennis serve, putting something on a high shelf, or an occasional home-improvement project like painting the ceiling—the movement of your arms takes your ribs with them. Your shoulder has adapted to what you do most frequently, but what you do most frequently is not what's best for your shoulder, or for the abdominal muscles that are displaced when you go to use your arms.

Were you living in an earlier time—when food and water were not readily available, let alone less than three feet from you at all times—your body would be adapted to a much wider range of movements. Your body would be stronger. Your body would not be collapsing.

Modern living does not require that we move, and to add insult to injury, it actually limits full use of our body. For example, a couch, although super comfortable, limits the full use of your ankles, knees, and hips. It sets the distance over which your leg and hip muscles can work. If you're leaning against something right now, that something is doing the work your core muscles would be doing were that thing not there. We've effectively outsourced the use of our bodies to our stuff. And then when we ask our bodies to hold us up, and hold stuff in, they fail. Make no mistake, it's not only the tissue that's broken; it's the habitat.

The most accurate answer to the question, "What created my diastasis recti?" is, "Your diastasis recti was created when the forces applied to your linea alba deformed it." But I know that's a biomechanist kind of answer and not really the answer you're after. So, taking a step back: your body wasn't strong enough to handle the loads placed upon it. Okay, there's a simple solution for that. There are exercises to do and movements to add that can improve the strength and the balance of strength throughout your body. And now, taking another step back: your habitat is shaping your body and loading your linea alba when you're not moving. This, too, is simple enough to remedy. We can change our shoes, our relationship with furniture, and how we set up our home and work environment. Don't worry, I'm not going to tell you to throw out all the stuff in your current life. What I will do is help you discover the best in both your habitat and your body.

NUTRITIOUS MOVEMENT

Let's talk food for a minute. Say that you eat a particular diet for a few years, but over that time fail to consume all of the essential dietary nutrients. You've missed something—you didn't eat enough protein, or you didn't eat enough vitamin D. Say you develop a particular health problem, so you head off to your nutritionist who, after reviewing your diet journal, quickly finds that your ailment is a known side effect of missing nutrient X. You replace the missing nutrient and, bam, no more ailment.

When it comes to ailments brought about by how you've moved, the process is very much the same. Movement—the constant changing of your orientation to gravity—supports various biological functions via the push and pull of working muscles. Therefore, when we have a musculoskeletal ailment of the body, it's prudent to first check that are we getting our essential movement nutrients.

WHAT ARE THE MOVEMENT NUTRIENTS?

Every motion you make with your body—from standing still to hopping log to log and from taking a walk to taking a breath—uses your core. And so, your core can only be as strong as the moves you cycle through each day, as well as the quality of those moves. If you don't move that much, or don't move that well, your core will continue to be a weak link for you.

I like to break down movement into macronutrients (large categories of movements) and micronutrients (isolated moves, or "corrective exercises," that assist you in assessing and then refining the quality of your larger motions). The macronutrients of human movement include:

- Walking
- Squatting and Floor-sitting (unsupported resting)
- Lifting/Carrying
- Hanging/Swinging/Climbing

Micronutrients, then, are exercises that help enable you to walk or squat or carry something in a way that uses your body better.

Under conventional treatment, at worst, you might be told there is no solution to your diastasis recti besides surgery. And at best, you might be given a corrective exercise program by a trained therapist. Treating a diastasis recti with corrective exercise is similar to treating most ailments arising from a muscular imbalance. Corrective exercises are most often used in the same way vitamins and minerals are—as supplements to fill a void. Your left gluteus doesn't fire when you walk, so your hip twists more on one side? That twist creates a small tug on the linea alba, which wears it out more on one side, and thus creates tissue damage there. Vitamin "Gluteus Exercise" for you! (Take twelve, three times a day, and call me in the morning.)

This approach works for some, yet many people I know, therapists and patients alike, spend their entire life solving one problem—and then another, and then another.

At some point, we have to look at our bottles (programs, books, videos) of supplements (corrective exercises and equipment) and ask ourselves, "What's wrong with this picture?" Is our understanding of movement nutrition so far off that we spend the bulk of our time seeking the best supplements rather than the best diet? Have we really decided that the solution to our musculoskeletal ailments is a lifelong program that consists of running through our list of corrective exercises for our abs, our weak shoulder, our trick knee? Or at some point would we like to learn how to use our bodies in a way that requires no supplemental exercise? Do you want to learn how to set up your life so that *the way you execute your daily living* is more nutritious for your body—no extra time required?

FLAT ABS ARE NOT NECESSARILY DIASTASIS RECTI–FREE ABS

Many women, especially after giving birth, feel that the lack of flatness in their abdomen is the indicator for diastasis recti, and begin to associate abdominal flatness with abdominal closure (i.e., bringing the two parts of the rectus abdominis back together again). This logic poses a problem. There are many flat-stomached fitness professionals that have a diastasis recti, and getting your abdominal muscles closer to the midline does not a flat belly make. There are also many people without a diastasis recti sporting fat on their midsection. One fascinating study (check out Brauman, 2005 in the references) showed that, in the observation of patients seeking an abdominoplasty (tummy tuck), the greatest protrusion of the abdomen did not line up with the area of the widest diastasis. My motivation for writing this book is to assist you in finding the strongest, most functional version of your body possible, which includes high-functioning abs as noted by how they function (movement tests) rather than how they look—which can be misleading.

In Section 2, you will absolutely find corrective exercises. I teach (and use, personally) corrective exercise every day. But. BUT. In the last five years I have transitioned to a more nutritious movement diet—a way of moving through my life—that has kept me from needing copious amounts of movement supplements in the form of exercise. So, in Section 2 you will also find the non-exercise, day-to-day adjustments to how you live that directly translate to a better mechanical environment for your core muscles.

Eventually you can transition to a more nutritious movement diet, and this book is a great start.

Are you ready to learn how to move for a high-functioning core that is strong and supports you and all your amazing biological processes? Say it with me: "YES, I AM."

Fantastic. It's time for Section 2.

KEY POINTS:

- Diastasis recti is a symptom of how you've moved your entire body throughout your entire life. There may have been a "straw that broke the camel's back," but it really is a whole-body, whole-life issue.

- Corrective exercises ("micronutrients") can serve as vitamins and minerals to nourish under- or over-moved areas, but in the same way you can't live on minerals and vitamins (you must eat food), corrective exercises cannot fully meet the "movement nutrition" requirements of your body.

- Corrective exercises done in conjunction with or to help you execute the movement macronutrients will result in a stronger, more robust body that has a stable midsection. Like the carpet spot that stops fading when you block out the damage-inducing light, a torso used dynamically will "block out" the weakness because it is functional enough to do so.

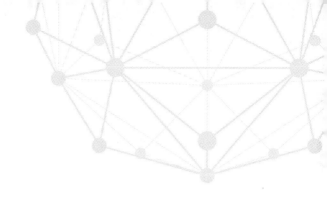

SECTION 2: MOVE

EQUIPMENT LIST
Here are all the items you'll need for the upcoming section.
Wherever possible, I list alternatives to "official" equipment. In
most cases, you'll have the items you need in your house and
won't need to purchase any additional equipment!

- bolster (and/or blankets, towels, pillows)
- chair
- log (or other longish, weighted item)
- resistance band (or pair of tights)
- yoga block (or stack of folded towels)
- yoga mat (or other soft surface, like a carpet)
- yoga strap (or belt, rope, etc.)

Optional tools for self-myofascial release exercises (page 151)

- large exercise ball
- Yoga Tune Up® Coregeous® ball (or another very soft, pliable, medium-sized ball)
- tennis ball (or a Pinky ball, or Yoga Tune Up® ball)

The "best" exercise prescription
Movement science is in its infancy, and so the best "dosage"
of various exercises isn't known yet. I'll occasionally give notes
about how long to hold certain positions, or how many times
to do an exercise, but the ideal we are really after is for you
to be able to do these movements as often as you can while
maintaining good form. This is the best way to elicit adaptation.

STANCE AND
"BODY NEUTRAL"

CHAPTER 5

I have a brother who is both a smoker and an endurance runner—activities he swears cancel each other out, like adding 3 and -3 gets you 0. As you can imagine, I disagree.

The opposite of smoking isn't running, it's *not smoking*, and while running can absolutely increase the performance of the lungs, endurance training does not undo the damage to the lungs caused by smoking. Still, much of the world truly believes that the corrective for a health issue (lung problems, for my brother) is not to change the environment in which it occurred (i.e., smoking), but to add something (like running) on top of the habits that led to the issue and hope for a different net outcome.

I don't like to give corrective exercises without context— without a larger goal of moving better as a lifestyle. Without this context, "corrective exercises" can perpetuate the idea that there are in fact exercises that offset poor movement habits. You won't lose weight by eating a Snickers bar and then eating a salad to offset the Snickers. Both go into the body and do what they do. A Snickers isn't undone simply because you've made a better food choice before or after eating it. A salad isn't "corrective eating." And you can't offset sitting all day and not using your core by doing a handful of exercises. You are still putting a ton of non-movement into your body, which adapts to that non-movement input as much as to the movement input.

For the best results and lasting improvement, you must change the habits that led to the issue in the first place. I suggest you think of corrective exercises as the first steps towards changing how you use your body all of the time—not just when you're doing the exercises. There is no list of exercises that will repair your DR, but there is, I have found, a list of exercises that, when combined with altering how you sit, stand, get up, get down, and move with your body all day long, result in success.

Balancing your body—establishing a physiological and mechanical homeostasis—requires a broad use of your body. Just as we've been told to "eat the rainbow" to gather a wide spectrum of dietary nutrients, we must move in multiple ways if we're to strengthen our core relative to our upper body and lower body, and stay strong enough to handle loads created by the complex movements life throws at us. To make sure you're getting a little movement in each category, let's revisit my list of movement macronutrients. It's important to be competent in moving in each of these ways:

- Walking
- Squatting and Floor-sitting (unsupported resting)
- Lifting/Carrying
- Hanging/Swinging/Climbing

Each of these categories of movement uses the core muscles in a different way—which is why moving lots of different ways is like eating a variety of foods. Each food (I mean, movement) nourishes your core differently.

If you want a strong and dynamic core, then you've got to use it in challenging ways. But when the connection between your muscles has been compromised—as it has in the case of a DR—executing the macronutrients in a way that restores your core can be difficult. This is where the micronutrients—the smaller motions found in my corrective exercises—come into play.

The following sections include corrective exercises designed to mobilize and strengthen the commonly underused and/or overly tense parts of you that can lead to a DR, as well as habit modifications to help you change how you sit, stand, get up, get down, walk, and even *get dressed* in the morning. These corrective exercises are like the running my brother does for better lung function, and the habit modifications are to assist you in "not smoking," meaning they will stop the all-day loads that created a DR in the first place.

You should find that the exercises and habit modifications reinforce each other—the more you do the correctives, the more easily you'll be able to stand and sit and move in a way that uses your abdomen all day long, and the more you use your muscles naturally throughout the day, the less you'll need the correctives. Your body—especially your trunk—will become stronger from the way you use it in day-to-day life.

YOUR FEET ARE THE FOUNDATION OF YOUR CORE

Most exercises in this book require unshod feet—or at least shoes without a heel. A heeled shoe forces a change in the geometry of your ankle joint, which in turn forces a change at the knees, which forces a change at the hips and to the tilt of your pelvis, which forces a change in the position of your ribcage, all of which alters the length and force-production capability of your core muscles. It's not rocket science; it's geometry: how you stand sets the stage for how your abdominal muscles are able to function, and what you wear on your feet affects how you stand. Wearing a shoe with *any* amount of heel changes the load to the linea alba. Specifically, heels require that you adjust your pelvic tilt or ribcage position to compensate for the height under the heel bone of your foot.

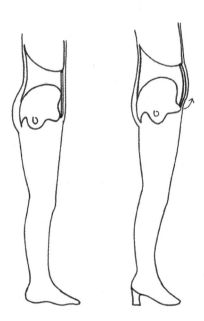

Check out your shoe closet (and your kid's too, if you have one). Is there a raised heel on just about every shoe you own? I'd be willing to bet there's been a heel on almost every shoe you've worn every day of your life. And, if you've been following what I've said so far—that how you move all day has more of an impact on your abdomen than exercises do—then you'll know why I suggest transitioning to having bare feet or minimalist shoes most of the time.

Like a fantastic dessert at a special occasion dinner, a heeled shoe is no biggie now and then, but because you've been wearing heels of many shapes the bulk of your life, your abdominal muscles and the tension on your linea alba have been affected. How they've been affected depends on your size and shape and what other movements you have (or haven't) done throughout your life, but setting all that uniqueness aside, until your trunk is healed, it's best to stay out of a heel as much as possible.

(If you need more details about the ways in which a heeled shoe affects your alignment, or how to transition safely to wearing minimalist shoes all the time, read *Whole Body Barefoot*. Or you can just take my word for it, and find yourself some completely flat shoes.)

It's not only your shoes knocking your abs off-kilter—as I discussed briefly, the position of your legs and pelvis can also change the loads to the linea alba. Ballet and military training both start with lessons in position so that certain positions can be called upon at a moment's notice. We'll start in a similar way, by learning a sort of "body neutral" position I can refer you back to over and over again. You can also assume full or partial body neutral when you're standing around in line or as you move through the exercises I recommend.

BODY NEUTRAL
·······························

▸ FEET PELVIS-WIDTH APART

Standing in front of a mirror, line up the middle of the front of your ankles with the bony prominences at the front of your pelvis (called your anterior superior iliac spines or ASIS).

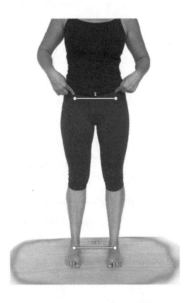

This better distributes the weight of the body over the entirety of both knees. This arrangement is easier to do when standing still than while walking, but even widening your ankles slightly makes a difference. If, for example, you tend to walk with your ankles very close together—similar to walking on a tightrope—open them just a bit, bringing the ankles closer to pelvis-width apart. This new position sets you up with a better geometry for using the muscles in your hips once you start walking.

▸ BACK YOUR HIPS UP (AND TAKE A LOAD OFF YOUR LINEA ALBA)

If you stand sideways to a mirror, and hang a plumb line down from the center of your hip joint, you'll probably find that the other end is dangling over the front of your foot.

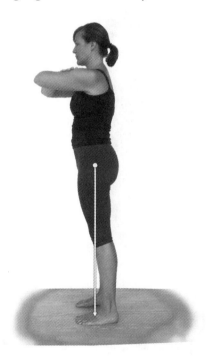

The loads created by standing this way are problematic for many reasons, but setting aside things like increased psoas tension, lower-back compression, and reduced weight-bearing status of the hips, this particular body geometry increases the tension on the linea alba—both in the top-to-bottom and in the side-to-side directions.

To correct this pelvic thrust, move your hips back so that they're directly over the knees and ankles—so that the plumb line picks up the midpoint of the knee and the quarter-sized ankle bone over the heel.

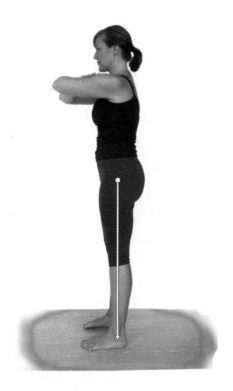

You might find that you don't have the strength to stand with vertical legs at first, but the more you back up (and stop wearing heels that prevent you from standing with a vertical leg), the more you will use—and develop—your glutes and hamstrings to hold you upright.

▶ NEUTRAL FEMURS

Our legs aren't just poky things that stick out of our hips; they're connected to the pelvis with muscles—muscles that can change the position of your pelvis and thus the load to the linea alba.

Start by pointing your feet straight ahead, so that the lateral malleoli (the outer quarter-sized ankle bone) is in line with the bony prominence just behind the pinkie toe. (I know, it feels weird, but eventually you will want to end up walking with your feet straight like this all the time. Make the change gradually, decreasing the amount your feet turn out a little bit at a time, until you end up feeling comfortable with your feet pointing straight.)

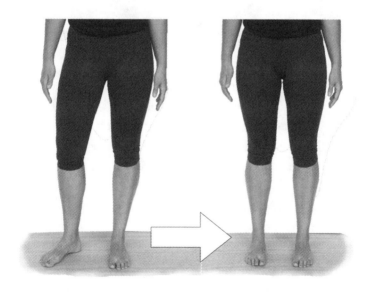

Standing with a mirror (or a close friend) behind you, turn your thighbones (femurs) outward until the four lines down the back of both knees line up like this:

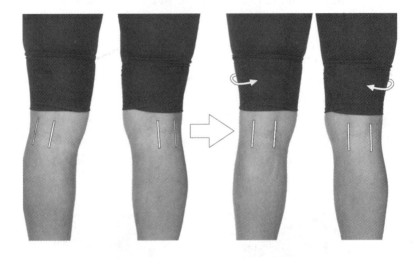

Note that the degree to which you need to rotate your femurs will depend on how much they've been rotated, and will probably vary between your two legs. Also important to note: you do NOT need to keep the instep of the foot down as you rotate your thighs to neutral. To do so can create a high torsional load to the knee, so instead let the inner edges of the feet lift away from the ground! (image next page)

I mentioned earlier that our chronic sitting and shoe-wearing has changed the geometry of our bodies, and in the case of this exercise, you're likely to find that years of underusing the thirty-three joints inside each foot has left your foot kind of clumped together as a single unit. It is this clumping that tends to rotate the thighs inward in the first place, which then tends

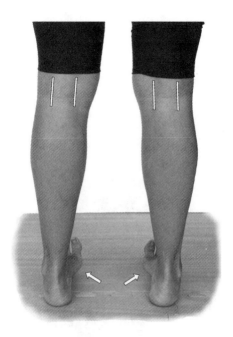

to turn off the muscles of the hamstrings and glutes when you're walking, which then leads to you thrusting your pelvis forward when you're standing at rest. You see? It's all connected. To help mobilize your feet so that you can stand and walk with better-aligned thighbones, which will help you have stronger muscles that keep the load off of the linea alba, work your feet over a tennis or therapy ball (and find out more about "feet straight" and intrinsic foot muscle mobilization exercises in *Whole Body Barefoot*).

▸ NEUTRAL PELVIS

The pelvis is made up of three bones—two iliac bones (one on the right and one on the left side), and a sacrum in the back. The anterior superior iliac spines (ASIS) are the most prominent anterior (front) superior (above) bony projections on the right and left sides of your pelvis. People often refer to these points as the hipbones (as in, "Put your hands on your hips"). The pubic symphysis is the joint at which the two hipbones come together. It is the lowest bony prominence before your pelvis wraps around to the undercarriage.

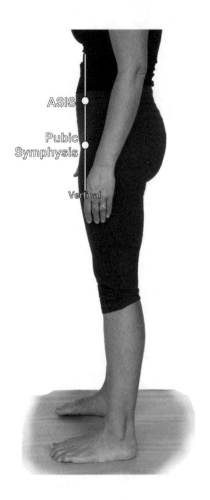

To find your pelvis's neutral position, arrange the ASIS and the pubic symphysis vertically.

If your hips and/or spine are really tight, you might find yourself tensing various muscles to achieve this position. This is where the corrective exercises (a.k.a. movement micronutrients) come in handy. When you mobilize these areas, your body should fall into alignment without you needing to force it. Remember, the forces you use to create a position are just as important as the position you've chosen, so straining to attain a neutral pelvis is really an indication that you need to do your correctives more often, as well as decrease any behaviors that are training your body away from the positioning you desire.

DROP YOUR RIBS

If I was going to make T-shirts to go with this book, they would say "DROP YOUR RIBS." Learning to better align your ribcage is crucial to improving the mechanical loads to your linea alba, because where your ribcage goes, it takes the linea alba with it. The body is capable of all sorts of movements, but it doesn't do sustained positions—especially those sustained for decades—very well.

To make a long story short, we lift our ribcage because the muscles of our chest, shoulders, and arms have adapted to desk work and minimal use, so that their resting position is slightly in front of the trunk. An easy correction *to the appearance* of a droopy chest is to lift it, and so "chest up and shoulders back" is just that—a quick adjustment for better appearance. Chest up, shoulders back changes how these parts align to the ground—now your upper body looks more upright—but it's done little to fix the issue of how the parts actually line up relative to each other. Your shoulders are still forward to your chest (your chest and shoulder muscles being weak and tight), only now you've compounded the problem by chronically pulling your ribcage away from your pelvis. The cue I use is "ribs down," but the corrective ribs-down motion isn't only lowering your ribs; rib lifting and lowering both create more complex motions on multiple planes.

Because of the hinge system of the spine and the muscles running between the pelvis and ribcage, lifting your chest swings the bottom of the ribcage forward while simultaneously tugging the right and left halves of the ribcage away from each other. This upward, forward, and expanding motion of the ribcage creates a load down the linea alba that's similar to the way unzipping a tight sweatshirt moves the right and left half of the sweatshirt away from each other.

It follows, then, that correcting the whole ribs up/ribs forward/ribs separated motion requires that you do the reverse—ribcage downward, backward, and…together.

That last part, "ribcage together," is the challenging part. While the lateral distancing of the ribcage is a passive motion—all you had to do was lift your chest to also thrust and separate your ribcage—the correcting of ribs apart needs to be more mindful. You can strengthen your "rib-closing" muscles (called the transversus thoracis) by doing the rib-closing exercises on page 92. Here's an even more effective method: Drop your ribs and back them up, aligning the torso, and then use your abdomen in a more dynamic and frequent way (see chapter 8 for larger "rib-closing" movements) that challenges your rectus abdominis to contract, drawing your ribs back together and strengthening your abdomen at the same time.

Although it's made of parts, your ribcage can be thought of as a single structure for this exercise. To find "neutral ribcage," rotate your ribcage down and back until the bottom front ribs align vertically with your ASIS and pubic symphysis.

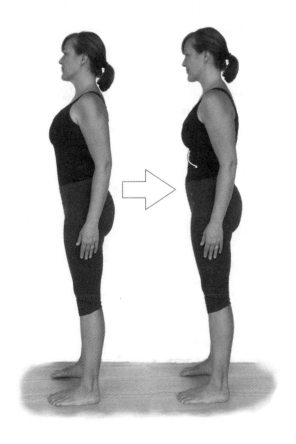

Now your torso is like a vertical tube, taking the tension off the linea alba, setting all your abdominal muscles up to respond to the motions you'll soon be creating. Aligning your ribcage also decreases compression of your spinal discs and vertebrae, and decreases the tension on any ligaments in your spine that have become lax due to repetitive hyperextension caused by rib-thrusting.

▶ RAPUNZEL, RAPUNZEL, LET DOWN YOUR DIAPHRAGM

If your torso were a building, it would have three storeys (your thoracic, abdominal, and pelvic cavities) and two floors (the diaphragm, between the thoracic and abdominal cavities, and the pelvic floor, below the pelvic cavity) (yes, it would be a kind of weird building, with no floor between the pelvic storey and the abdominal storey, but bear with me). When you hold in your stomach, the contents of your abdomen can be pressed up toward the diaphragm. This prevents your diaphragm from moving its full range of motion during breathing and it

DROPPING YOUR RIBS WHILE PREGNANT

Does it seem like you're decreasing the space available in your belly when you drop your ribs? Consider this: Lifting your ribs closes the back side of your container; dropping your ribs opens the back of the container up, keeping your abdominal volume consistent. By shifting the geometry of your container in this way, you not only maintain baby-space, you also decrease the stress on the linea alba (and pubic symphysis, incidentally), and position the uterus over the pelvis—leading to better uterine support.

negatively impacts the use of your abdominal muscles. I hate to be the one to tell you, but here I go: you're going to have to let your diaphragm down and the only way you can do that is to let out any belly that you're trying to hide in your abdominal cavity. There are two levels to this exercise, the first being the easiest on the linea alba.

Place your hands on your upper abdomen and allow your entire belly to relax, paying special attention to the sensation of your diaphragm releasing. You will probably feel your abdominal contents moving outward, both sensing the motion and feeling it with your hands. Once you feel you've released your diaphragm, try again—chances are you are holding residual tension there. You will likely need to remind yourself to relax your diaphragm throughout the day.

A more advanced version of the diaphragm release is to relax your belly to the floor while on your hands and knees. In this quadruped position, your abdominal contents rest their weight more on your linea alba than they do in the seated version, making the quadruped version of this exercise an important one later down the road, especially if you're doing other exercises on your hands and knees. If you always suck in your stomach when you're on your hands and knees, your abdominal muscles can't engage well.

I'd like to note that relaxing your diaphragm and letting out any fat you've been pulling inside your belly does not equal "turning your abs off." Muscles are always on; their job is to monitor the movements you're doing and respond accordingly. When you're sitting there in your chair, it's entirely natural for your stomach to soften. Why would these muscles be working? Your chair and your slouchy position are holding you, and you're

ON BREATHING

In order to breathe—to get air into your nose and down into your lungs—you have to drop the pressure within your thoracic cavity so that air flows in. By now, you're an expert on pressure, so you know that in order to drop the pressure you're going to have to increase the space (volume) within the thoracic cavity. Because the walls of this section of your body are mostly muscular, it's easy for you to change the shape (and thus volume) of your thoracic cavity. You can lower the diaphragm to make more space, flare your ribs open to make more space, or elevate your shoulders. You can do any combination of all three. In most cases, though, the muscles in our ribs and arms are stiff and unused and the diaphragm is typically locked in the UP position. As demonstrated so well by my horse Penny, many of us have developed ways to breathe while holding in the stomach and our body has adapted to those ways. This is a long way of saying that many people find it difficult to breathe when they release their diaphragm.

It totally messes with your breathing game, changing up the geometry of your body parts. When you couple it with shoulders and ribcage muscles gone stiff from a lifetime of desk and computer work, trying to breathe in your new position can cause downright panic. So. Step one is to keep breathing. DID I MENTION YOU SHOULD KEEP BREATHING? If you notice you're having trouble breathing with your diaphragm released, go back to the position where breathing is comfortable. Then, check in with your ribs—they need to be all the way down in order to take over the work of breathing. If that still doesn't help, forget the diaphragm release for now and work on the rib dropping and corrective exercises for awhile; then circle back to try it again.

not moving. There's no reason for your abdominal muscles to be working when you sit in a chair!

Because we sit so much, we modern humans have developed a correction for naturally non-working abs: we train ourselves to tense them all the time. We don't get up and move more so that our abdominals can respond to what we're doing; we stay seated and fake core use through tension. Unfortunately, the faking doesn't cut it, because the only ab movement we can fake is static tension, and tension in the abdominals does not help out a diastasis recti. In fact, it can make it worse.

You want the muscles in your midsection to be working all the time, but to get them to fire naturally, you've got to get moving.

STANCE: CHECK IT OUT

Pilots use checklists to ensure they don't forget essential tasks along the way, and since you are essentially piloting your body, it is helpful to keep a note at your computer desk (or any place you find yourself with regularity) reminding you to:
- Straighten your feet
- Back your hips up
- Align your knee pits
- Adjust your pelvis
- Drop your ribs
- Relax your diaphragm

It seems like it should be easy—just putting your body where you want it to be—but many of these adjustments require better strength and the mobility of smaller, under--utilized muscles.

LITTLE MOVES

CHAPTER 6

So you want to restore your core—that's great (and so catchy we considered it for the title of this book). But in order to do that, you have to know what the function of the core is. If you don't know what your core *should* be doing, then how can you know when you've fixed it?

In *Move Your DNA* I likened the abdomen to a tennis player. A tennis player's job is to win the game, and in order to do that, the player needs to be able to respond appropriately to any shot that comes his way. Your abdomen's job is to perform optimally. On one hand you can think of "optimal" as looking fierce in your bathing suit or being able to do a thousand crunches without stopping. On the other hand, you could consider the biological functions that occur within your trunk, like the distribution of blood and oxygen throughout your body (the cardiovascular system), the digestion and elimination of food (the digestive system), supporting and delivering a baby (the reproductive system), and the freedom to move without pain. This book is about the latter, biological definition of optimal—where the successes of your body's basic physiological processes are used as an indication of how your body is doing physically.

In addition to knowing what kind of core outcomes you can be looking for, consider what the core muscles themselves do.

Core muscles flex, twist, bend, and stabilize the spine. They also provide the connection between your upper and lower body. They can carry the weight of your lower half up toward your upper half as you're moving down a set of monkey bars. They can haul your legs up to something you're hanging on to.

When you think of the variety of tasks the core muscles should be capable of, the inadequacies of common core training programs quickly become apparent. Many people end their core training program at the same place they began—the same handful of exercises, performed with low amounts of body weight, at a high repetition. Your core can do more, and it must in order for you to keep it strong and supple.

If you compare your use of abdominal muscle to what your abdominal muscles are capable of, you'll soon find out why your dream midsection is eluding you. Core function is based on use, and it's time you used your core well—and reaped both the biological and the aesthetic rewards.

GETTING TO THE CORE OF THE CORE

I know, that last section sounded like I was gearing up to drill-sergeant you into shape, but relax. Your kick-a$$ abdominal routine is going to start with…small stretches. Actually, it's going to feel like stretching, but what you'll really be doing is moving subtly, in new ways, while busting up fused areas of your body so that you can get to the more challenging stuff. Which isn't to say the correctives are going to be easy—only that they will be gentle on your body. (And by the time you get to the BIG MOVES section, you'll likely find that those "hard moves" you thought you weren't *strong* enough to do were actually hard because your body wasn't *mobile* enough to capitalize on the geometry that makes them doable.)

FREEING UP YOUR UPPER BODY

Here's why we're starting with the upper body: your shoulders are probably wicked tight, wicked weak, or both. Remember, your abdominal muscles *should* be working, in some way, to some extent, every time you move. Our arms, though, have adapted to little use and highly repetitive positioning, and whenever we go to use them, they pull the ribs with them—displacing the abdominal muscles and tugging on the linea alba. In order to be able to use our trunk muscles while doing more dynamic movements like carrying kids or groceries, doing pull-ups at the gym, or swinging down a set of monkey bars, we must be able to separate the arms from the ribcage, so that we can keep our ribs down and abdominal muscles working no matter what our arms are doing.

BOLSTERS ARE YOUR NEW BFF

Coming up are many lying-down exercises to help you separate the arms from the ribcage, and the ribcage from the pelvis. But because our upper spines have sort of collapsed due to a general lack of physical strength, it's extremely likely that when you lie down on your back your ribs push away from the floor. Which means **the very act of lying on your back can be reinforcing the forces that create a DR**. Until your body is more mobile, use the following bolstering technique when performing all floor exercises.

You can use a bolster, blankets, towels, and/or pillows to support your head and upper spine—wherever they may be—once your legs are extended (with the backs of the hamstrings, the muscles on the back of the thigh, touching the floor) and your ribs are down in neutral.

The easiest way to do this is to lie down on your back with your legs out in front of you (remember, aim for the backs of the thighs to be touching the ground), with your pile of bolstering goodies to one side. Using your arms to support you as you move, do a "crunch" motion of the torso, stopping when the ribcage is aligned with the pelvis and you're no longer thrusting.

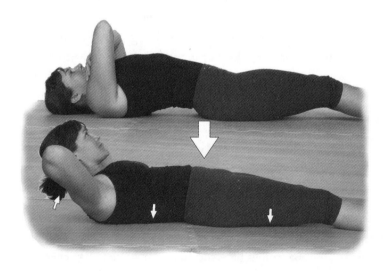

This "crunch" is the same rib-lowering motion you do when standing and correcting your rib-thrust, only when you're lying on the ground you're working against gravity instead of with it. (We use our elbows to hold up our body weight so as not to create any unnecessary downward pressure, which can overload the core when it's in a weakened state.)

Fill the gap between your head, shoulders, and the ground with bolsters (again, these could be blankets, yoga bolsters, pillows, etc.) until your ribs-down position is fully supported and your abdomen is in neutral, but not working to maintain its neutrality.

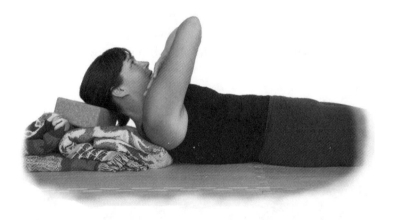

Throughout this exercise section I'll keep reminding you to **bolster your torso** to keep your ribs down as necessary.

SMALL MOBILIZING EXERCISES

▶ FLOOR ANGELS

Begin by reclining on a bolster or stacked pillows so that your ribcage can lower toward the floor. Reach your arms out to the sides, keeping the palms facing up and the elbows lifting up toward the ceiling. Try to get the backs of your hands to the floor, **keeping your elbows slightly bent**. Once your chest can handle this stretch, slowly move your arms toward your head, only going as far as you can keeping your thumbs on the floor while trying to lift your elbows away from the floor.

Keep checking in with your ribcage, making sure that your ribs aren't coming along for the ride. Make a "snow angel" motion ten times, moving slowly and **making sure to not go any higher than what you can do with your ribs down on the ground.**

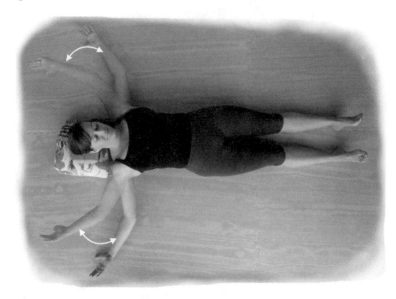

▸ WINDMILL STRETCH

Starting on your back, bring your right knee up toward your chest and then roll your entire body to the left, until your knee rests on the ground. (Note: This is not a spinal twist, where your ribs stay down and your pelvis rotates away from the upper half of the body, but your entire torso rolling to one side. You'll be doing a spinal twist in a while, but not yet.)

Check to make sure that, even in this rolled-over position, you're not thrusting your ribs.

Without hyperextending your elbow, reach your right hand, arm, and shoulder blade up toward the ceiling and away from the spine. Slowly drop your arm to the right as far as you can without thrusting your ribcage (it's okay if it doesn't go to the floor) until you find the boundary of your tension. Once there, imagine your arm is on the face of a clock. Keeping your palm facing the ceiling, slowly move your arm between twelve and six

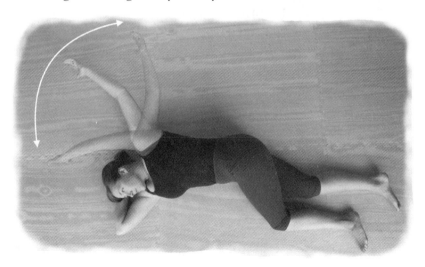

o'clock—up toward the head and straight out to the right and then down to your hip and then back up again.

(image previous page)

Do this 10–15 times, continuously reaching your elbow away from your torso (this keeps you from hyperextending your elbow) and checking that you're not thrusting your ribs!

Repeat on the other side.

▸ DOORWAY WALKTHROUGH

Each time you walk through a doorway is an opportunity to improve the relationship between your arm, rib, and core muscles. Reach your arms up until you can touch the wall above the doorway, and then drop your ribs back to neutral. Keeping the arms straight, step forward to increase the stretch, but really focus on…you guessed it…dropping your ribs. Play around with the position of your elbows (i.e., the rotation of the shoulder). Do they always point away from each other? Try a few with your elbows pointing straight ahead and see how movements of the shoulder change the load and the tendency to compensate with the ribs. (image next page)

And did I mention drop your ribs?

If you can, loop your fingers around an edge (i.e., a doorframe or a molding, if there is one) and lower your weight towards the floor, doing the bulk of the work with your legs but a smidge of work with your arms (a very gentle pre-cursor to the larger hanging exercise in the BIG MOVES chapter).

In the course of a day I walk through doorways at least a hundred times, which means these little twenty- to sixty-second doorway hangs break up my arm geometry with greater frequency than one fifteen-minute hanging session does.

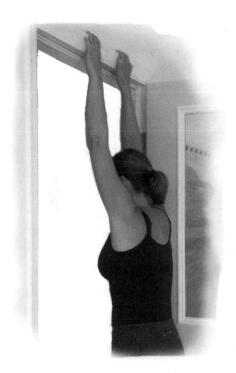

If you find yourself unable to reach the top of a doorway, you can do a single-armed version of this exercise, doing one arm at a time on the right and then left side of a doorway.

SMALL STRENGTHENING EXERCISES

The only reason I'm calling these exercises "small" is because the loads placed on the body are low, making them excellent moves to train your body to move better. These exercises, like the ones above, challenge your abdominal muscles to work relative to moving arms, moving ribs, and to a moving pelvis.

▸ LOG PULLOVER

I call this exercise the Log Pullover because I figure most people can get their hands on a log (one that would fit easily into a fireplace and doesn't weigh more than ten pounds). You can also do this exercise with any long, slightly weighted object.

Start the Pullover by lying on your back with your legs extended on the floor. Grip the ends of a log and squeeze your elbows toward each other (tight shoulders may make them want to poke out to the right and left). Keeping the ribs down, lower the log overhead, only going as far as you can without letting your ribs lift up toward the ceiling, then bring it back to the starting position. Repeat fifteen to twenty times.

I certainly didn't invent pullover exercises—you can find them being done in most gyms across the world. That said, I typically see them being done with a rib-thrusting motion (see image below; somebody forgot to bolster!), where the ribcage is moving up and down on a vertebral hinge, or with elbows dropping out to the sides (internal rotation of the shoulder). In both of these cases, the loads to the abdominals and the shoulder muscles are reduced, rib-thrusting habits are promoted, and the loads to spinal ligaments and the linea alba are high.

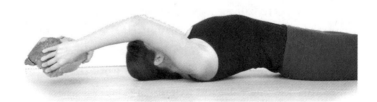

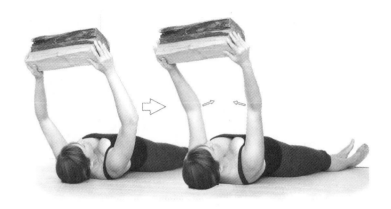

When you first begin this exercise, you'll likely need to keep your ribs bolstered in order to have them to stay neutral to the pelvis.

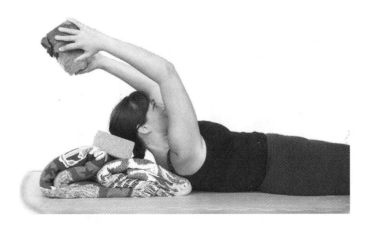

This will keep the exercise focused on mobilizing the arms from the ribcage. As your shoulders become more mobile, you can remove the bolstering and use this same exercise as an abdominal strengthener—using your rectus abdominis (instead of the bolster) to stabilize the ribcage.

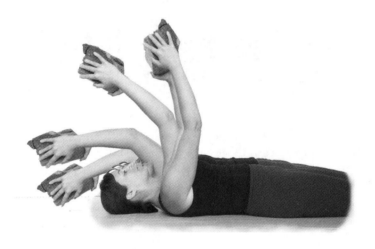

If you pay attention to the exercise you'll find that as the log drops farther away from you, the abdominals have to work more, and as the log moves closer to the knees, you'll be working your core less. By allowing your abdominals to respond according the load—more when the load is high and less when the load is small—you'll be varying the work of your abdominals. You'll note that this is a different instruction from "keep your ribs pressed to the ground," which would engage your stomach muscles to a degree that had nothing to do with the overhead motion; you would develop an excessive amount of tension in your abdomen instead of training it to respond naturally and dynamically—that is, how your abdominal muscles work best.

If you ditch the bolster and find that you are struggling to keep your ribs down throughout the motion, the log might be too heavy for your current capability. Go get some kindling and try it again.

STRENGTHEN YOUR RIBCAGE

While there isn't a right way to breathe, there are muscle tensions and weaknesses that render useless parts of the body that should be participating regularly in breathing. In between each rib is a group of muscles (called intercostals) that can move the rib up and down, increasing the size (volume) of the ribcage and creating a flow of air into the lungs. When your ribs don't move—and oftentimes they don't—you're still breathing (TELL ME YOU'RE STILL BREATHING!), but the diaphragm and the muscles of the shoulders have to work overtime to compensate for a lot of parts that are sitting there just taking a vacation. And those vacationing muscles in between the ribs? They're getting weaker and weaker. This exercise is to help you work the muscles in between the ribs, and there are a couple of reasons to do that. The first is that breathing is awesome and all of your breath-assisting muscles should be working. Another reason is that the less mobile your ribcage, the more you might be inflating the belly with each breath. Belly breathing is fine, but when you inflate your abdomen because your diaphragm has to move more to compensate for ribs that don't move, your belly breathing can come with a heavy load to tissues of the abdominal wall. This is also the exercise I use to bring the front of the right and left halves of the ribcage toward the midline, as mentioned on page 72.

▸ ACTIVATE YOUR INTERCOSTALS

Seated or standing, firmly tie a resistance band or pair of tights around your torso just beneath your chest muscles or breasts (at the height of a bra strap or heart rate monitor). Make sure you've dropped your ribs!

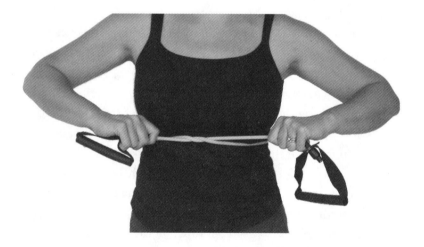

Inhale deeply, expanding the ribcage into the band until you feel the resistance from the elastic pushing on your ribs. If you don't feel it at the end of your inhale, re-tie the band and try it again.

Exhale, being aware of how your ribcage can pull away from the ring of elastic and closer to an imaginary vertical pole running up through the center of your body. Repeat, using each exhale to bring the ribs inward.

You should find (feel!) that breathing, especially the exhale, engages the muscles between the ribs and throughout the abdomen. You can use the elastic to teach you how to find and use these muscles, but once you've got the motor skill, you can do this exercise without the tactile assistance of the band.

FREEING UP YOUR WAIST

The above exercises were designed to generate better motion between the arms, ribs, and ribcage. This next set of exercises is designed to create better motion between the ribcage and the pelvis.

▸ FLOOR CRESCENT

Lying on your back, interlace your fingers and reach your arms overhead until your wrists touch the ground. You can probably guess what I'm going to say next. Did you guess? You're right. BOLSTER YOUR UPPER BODY UNTIL YOUR RIBS ARE DOWN. (see image next page)

Once your ribs are down, walk your arms and legs to the right as far as possible, keeping all four limbs on the floor. If your shoulders are tight, keeping the arms on the ground might cause the ribs to pop up. If this happens, modify by allowing the arms to come up as necessary. To start to work at tight waist/ hip muscles, cross your left ankle over your right to increase the stretch. You can also practice your intercostal activation breathing while holding this stretch for a minute or so. Repeat on the other side.

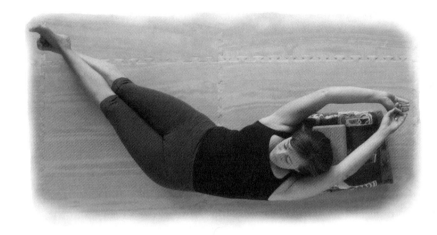

▸ SEATED SPINAL TWIST

The spinal twist is typically contraindicated for diastasis recti, as it can shear the right and left rectus abdominis away from each other. However, twisting is a natural motion that is required for everyday tasks, like checking over your shoulder when reversing your car. Also, the muscles of your waist are likely to be stiff and tense and constantly tugging your DR open. The only way to reduce that force is to get the waist supple and working; twisting is what the waist does, so we cannot avoid this motion—we can only learn how to do it well and in a way that serves the body.

Sit in a chair with a neutral pelvis and your ribs down (see page 135 for more information on how to align your sitting). Without jutting your ribs or tucking or untucking your pelvis, turn to the right and to the left without straining. Move to the edge of your range of motion, **taking care that you're not slightly moving out of alignment to go farther.**

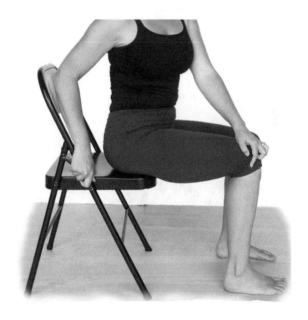

Once you've done this a few times, hold to one side, practicing the active intercostal exhale for 5 breaths. Then twist back and forth a few times and hold the twist to the other side (ribs down), doing the active intercostal exhale again, for 5 breaths. Complete the circuit with a few twists back and forth. **There are no points for speed**—the idea here is to become aware of your tendency to thrust your ribs (tugging on your linea alba) when your waist is tight, and to gain mobility in the obliques themselves.

▸ BOLSTERED SPINAL TWIST

As you can imagine, a DR-friendly on-the-floor spinal twist requires you to BOLSTER YOUR UPPER BODY UNTIL YOUR RIBS ARE DOWN. Did that read like I was shouting? I am. Bolster. Your. Ribs. Down.

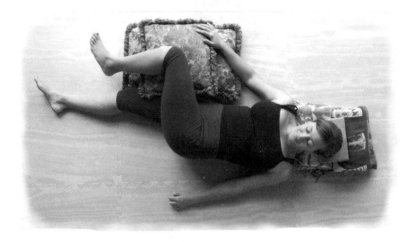

Once you're bolstered, scoot your pelvis an inch or two to the left, then bring the left knee up so that it stacks over your hip, and rotate your pelvis to lower that knee to the opposite side of your body, **stopping as soon as your ribs start to leave the ground**.

Most people, when they do a spinal twist, aren't twisting the spine; they're rolling the entire spine to one side. That's fine, unless they're trying to improve the mobility between the ribs and pelvis, in which case a spinal roll will get them nowhere... besides over to one side.

The goal in this spinal twist is not to force your knee to the floor but to note where your pelvis stops moving due to the tension in the trunk muscles. Twist only as far as you can without taking the ribs with you—no forcing it. This ensures that you'll stay on the edge of the boundary set by your current abdominal muscle tension. If you couple "ribs down" with "respecting your boundaries," this move won't be tugging on the linea alba.

If you find that your pelvis barely moves—if your trunk is that tight—and your knee is nowhere near the floor, you might want to **stack pillows so that the knee crossing over can rest on them.** This will reduce the load to the spine and keep these muscles from tensing unnecessarily.

Repeat on the other side.

▸ RIB SLIDE ON THE WALL

The good news is, you'll be a better dancer if you can master this next move. The bad news is, it might take a while, so feel free to do it when no one else is watching. Stand against a wall with your feet spread a bit wider than pelvis width, and get yourself lined up so that, while your feet remain a few inches from the wall, your bottom (no tucking the pelvis!) and your bra strap (or bro strap, gentlemen) are on the wall, and your ribs are D-O-W-N.

I never get tired of telling you to keep your ribs down.

Anyhow, once you've got these parts against a wall, you're going to slide your ribs to the right and left, creating a horizontal movement that requires the muscles between the ribs and pelvis to loosen up.

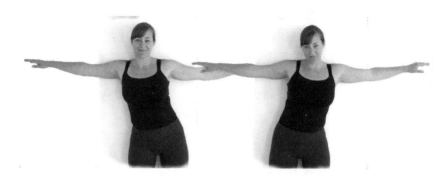

This motion is not as easy as it sounds, and **it is a common mistake to bend the torso to the right and left**, which is NOT the movement we are after here.

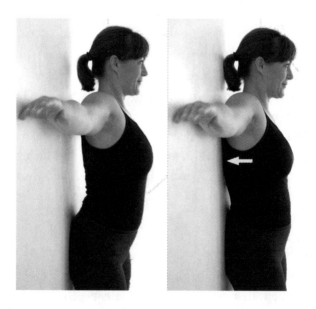

Ideally the shoulders and ribcage stay level as they move to the right and left of your pelvis.

Practice, practice, practice this until you can do it well, then head to the disco.

Note: Eventually you won't need a wall to do this exercise; the wall is only there to help you sense when you're twisting or thrusting away from the wall (see image previous page) instead of doing a purely side-to-side motion.

▸ CLICK-CLACK

This exercise is kind of challenging in that it's difficult to figure out which parts need to be moving and which need to be still. But stick with it; it is incredibly effective once you get the hang of it.

Start by sitting on the floor on a folded towel. You don't need a towel, but the towel will create a bolster that makes the motion easier to do at first.

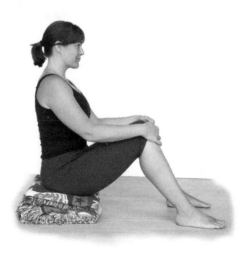

The Click-Clack motion is an anterior (forward) and posterior (backward) tipping motion of the pelvis. Before you start the exercise, see if you can tuck and untuck your pelvis.

Once you have some mobility, bend your knees until your feet are flat on the ground.

Holding on to your shins just below the knee, lean back until your arms are straight (**but not hyperextended),** and keep your ribs down.

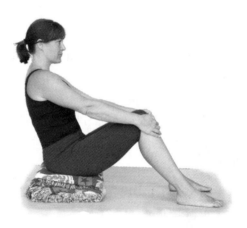

This is the Click-Clack position and it's important that you keep your body in this position (especially the straight arms and ribs down and feet down) throughout the exercise.

Without changing your arm length, tilt your pelvis forward and back, noticing the tendency to want to lift the chest. At first, your only job is to keep your arms straight and your ribs down while articulating only your pelvis.

Once this is easy for you, you need to begin paying attention to how you're getting your pelvis to tuck and untuck.

At first it's common to want to drive this motion by arching the back—to use the muscles in the spine to push your pelvis forward from behind it. But here's what I want you to do: I want you to steer the motion of your pelvis *with your feet*.

This is what you do: Keeping your feet in place (i.e., they're not going to go anywhere) push your feet away from you. At least, fire all the muscles you would if you wanted your feet to slide away from you—but don't let them. Firing those muscles while holding your feet in place will force the upper part of your pelvis behind you, rolling over your ischial tuberosities (sitting bones) and tucking your pelvis.

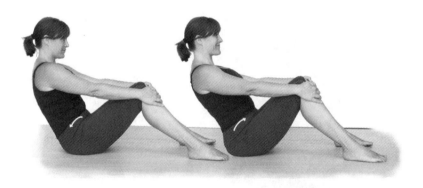

To get your pelvis to tilt forward, do the opposite foot work: try to draw your feet closer to you without letting them move and you'll rotate the top of your pelvis forward, creating an anterior (forward) tilt.

P.S. Why the name? I designed this exercise for my graduate work utilizing various exercises to correct pelvic floor disorder risk factors. When the participants first tried it, the action of rolling back and forth over their ischial tuberosities (the "sitting bones") created a loud thunking sound. Thus the study participants started calling this the Click-Clack and it stuck.

▶ DOORJAMB PULL-UP

Stand in a doorway and grasp the side of the doorway around shoulder height (as you practice you should vary the height at which you place your arm). Keeping your body vertical, your feet together and close to the wall, and your elbow pointing down to the floor (and not behind you), lower your body away from the doorway, and then pull yourself back up.

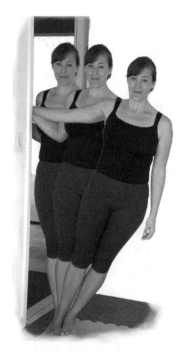

As your vertical torso moves into a diagonal position, more work is required of your core. And there's bonus arm work as well. To make the motion less difficult, move your feet away from the wall and start there, moving your feet toward the wall as you get stronger.

One common cheat is to let the hips drop away from and toward the wall (i.e.,

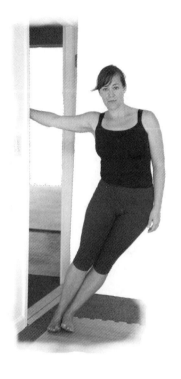

not keeping the body in a straight line throughout the move as in the "don't" image to the left).

Your core muscles are the ones working to keep your body straight, so the less straight your body, the less core work you'll be doing.

▸ **WALL CRESCENT**

Stand against a wall and get yourself lined up so that, while your feet remain a few inches from the wall, your butt, ribcage, and the back of your head are on the wall. Now, reach your arms over your head until your hands touch the wall above.

You might find that, keeping your ribs down, you aren't able to get your head or arms up against the wall. That's okay—it's more important for you to keep the legs straight, pelvis neutral, and ribs down than it is for you to touch the wall with your hands or head. The more you do this, the closer you'll be.

Now do a side bend, **without any twisting or thrusting**, using the wall as a guide to tell you when you have lost your alignment points. (image next page)

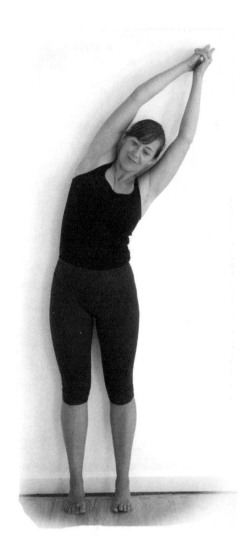

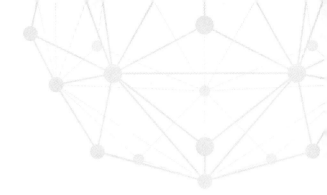

MEDIUM MOVES

CHAPTER 7

Medium moves are either slightly more challenging or use slightly larger and/or heavier body parts, like your legs. I'm listing the medium moves in order of difficulty, with the more gentle "stretching" type exercises first and the strength moves after those.

The idea with these exercises is the same as in the last chapter: to increase the mobility between the pelvis and the legs, and then strengthen the abdomen relative to the movements of your legs.

INNER THIGHS

We don't do much with our legs beyond walk to the next chair. Well, maybe we'll go for a run every now and then, but even then, we mostly use our legs in front-to-back motion, and hardly use any of the complex actions of our hips. This lack of complex use can leave the muscles of the inner thigh particularly weak, tight, stiff, and sore, and can over-connect the movements of the leg to the pelvis and vice versa.

The groups of muscles that form your inner thigh (their anatomical names are the adductors, medial hamstrings, and medial quadriceps) run between the pelvis and the thigh and/or the pelvis and your shin. When these muscles are tight, movements of your leg can carry the pelvis with them unnecessarily, sort of like a dysfunctional relationship can take you to places you weren't intending to go.

▸ **KNEE OUT TO THE SIDE**

Since we want to break up the motion between the thigh and the pelvis, we need to make sure that the pelvis doesn't move (much) during the next two exercises.

Lying face down with your belly on the floor, slide your left knee along the floor until it's out to your side, keeping your left

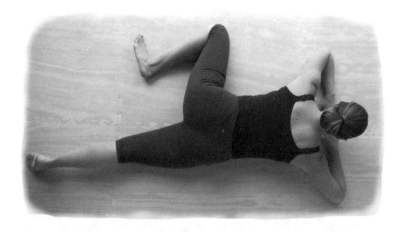

leg bent. If your hips are very stiff you might find that you can barely move the thigh at all without moving the pelvis. Don't fret. Turn your pelvis so that it "faces" the knee, and see if you can get the knee higher. Once it's closer to your head, turn the pelvis back to the floor, increasing the stretch. Hang out in the most comfortable place between knee up to the side and pelvis flat on the ground. You can be slightly uncomfortable with a stretching sensation, but **don't force your body into any position**. (image previous page)

Repeat on the other side, working up to a few times back and forth, holding each side about a minute.

▶ LEG OUT TO THE SIDE

Again, you'll be starting face down, and again, you'll be trying to (eventually) move your leg without moving your pelvis. Following the same rules as in Knee Out to the Side but with

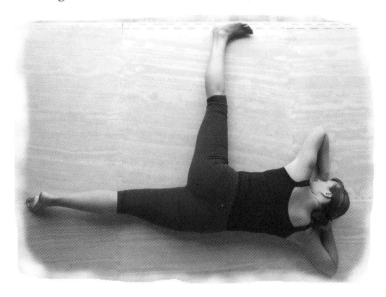

a straight leg, scoot your leg up toward your head, sliding it up along the floor. Bring it up as high as you can without lifting one side of the pelvis away from the floor or hiking one hip up toward your ribcage. A common cue I'll give when leading this exercise is: "keep the right and left sides of your waist the same length." (image previous page)

As you advance, try to externally rotate the stretching leg by rolling your thighbone so the toes on that foot point more toward the ceiling and less toward the floor. Rest your head and neck on your hands, hanging out here or in some modified position that allows you to relax.

▸ SUPINE SOLES TOGETHER

Lying on your back, bolstering the ribs as necessary, bend your knees until the soles of your feet are touching, then drop your knees out to the sides. If this is too much of a stretch for your

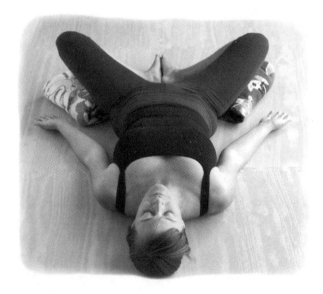

groin, **place pillows under each knee to support you in this position.** Lower the support bolsters as the position becomes more comfortable.

▶ SUPINE STACKED LEGS

Starting from the position of the last exercise, cross your ankles to place one ankle on top of the opposite shin. Let both knees drop toward the floor, **bolstering them as necessary.**

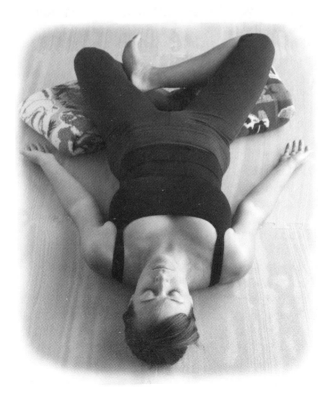

QUADRUPED

There are many exercises that can improve the overall function of your body that require what's called a quadruped position. Quadruped (*quad*, meaning four, and *ped*, meaning feet) is a fancy word for getting down onto your hands and knees. There are not many quadruped exercises in this book, but there are many quadruped exercises out there, and if you want to do them, here's a basic primer on how to make sure your quadruped is helping and not hurting your DR.

1. Begin on your hands and knees, relaxing your pelvis to neutral

Letting the pelvis untuck can be tricky when you have a DR, as you've probably developed the habit of tucking your pelvis under to pull your abdomen in. This is a short-term solution, since you've also displaced the attachments of your abdomen, preventing them from working well. The idea behind most quadruped exercises is to challenge your core, so if you're tucking, you're simply strengthening your coping mechanism (tucking) and not gaining better core function.

Compare the pictures on the opposite page and see if you can spot the tucked pelvis on the top.

2. Drop (I mean lift!) your ribs

Okay, so what I want you to do is align your ribs to your pelvis. It's the same rib-dropping motion you did while standing, only when you're on your hands and knees, it's really lifting your ribs back up toward the ceiling. However you need to think about it, get the ribs into neutral so that your abdominal wall is in the best geometrical position to sense the weight of your organs and respond appropriately.

When you then go to do the exercise, whatever it is—maybe you'll reach an arm out in front of you, or a leg out behind you—make sure you don't sacrifice the core's arrangement. **Watch in a mirror, keeping your eyes on your pelvis (don't let it tuck!) and your ribs (don't let them drop toward the floor).**

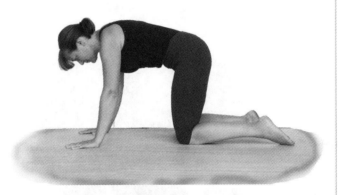

A tucked pelvis will create a flattened waistband area

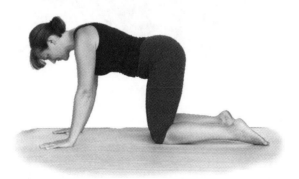

See the slight curve at the waistband?

▸ WIDE SQUAT WITH SIT-BACK

Starting on your hands and knees (don't forget to mind your ribs), widen your knees so they're wider than your pelvis. Then sit back toward your feet without tucking your pelvis. **Once your pelvis starts to tuck, STOP.** Pelvis tucking marks the end of your hips' range of motion, which is where you should be doing this exercise.

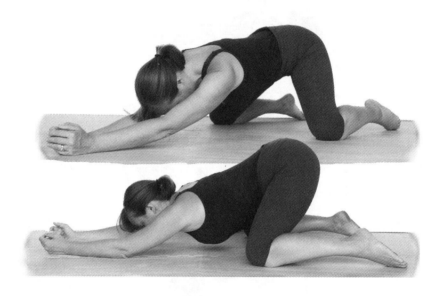

If you are very new to this motion and it is causing your body to tense or hurt, you can reduce the load by doing it on a bed or other soft or squishy surface, or **place one pillow or blanket behind your knees** (so they aren't forced into flexion), and one **under your ankles** (see image on next page) so that gravity doesn't force you beyond your current ranges of motion.

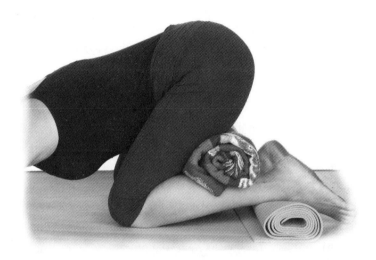

Once you're as far back as your pelvis can go without tucking, shift your pelvis from side to side, gently, to see if there's any tension deep in the hips. You can also do this exercise at different knee-widths; each width provides a different load!

FRONT OF THE THIGH

There are many muscles on the front of the thigh that connect the pelvis to the thigh and to the shin. These correctives are to help you break up any over-tense relationships.

▸ KNEECAP RELEASE

Try this: Stand up, unshod, paying attention to the tension in your feet and legs. Now move your hips forward. What you might notice is that as your weight moves forward, the tendency to topple forward increases. And so to balance out this new position, the front of the feet press into the ground (an isometric use of the "toe pointing" calf muscles) and the front of the thighs tighten, pulling your kneecaps upward (in the direction of your head).

Now you're going to learn how to relax your quads. Relaxing the quads sounds easy (after all, what's difficult about relaxing?!) but in the same way that calming down can be hard, so can dialing down your quad tension. If I said to you, "RELAX, MAN," chances are that relaxing would actually be challenging. Tension (like in the muscles that pull up the kneecaps) in many cases is not arbitrary but is instead a physiological coping mechanism for mechanical habits (like having stood with your pelvis out in front of you, over your toes, for a few decades).

I've taught the Kneecap Release for over a decade now and many find it frustrating. "IT'S SO SIMPLE, WHY CAN'T I DO IT?" While there may be more than one reason your kneecaps are still lifted, the easiest to explain is, "You're using your quadriceps muscles to keep from pitching forward."

Because you've likely been wearing heeled shoes and thrusting your pelvis throughout your entire life, and because you just learned how to back your pelvis up, give yourself some time to learn to relax the quads.

The instructions for this exercise, I hate to say it, are pretty simple. **Stand with your legs vertical** (as pictured on page 66) and let your kneecaps down by relaxing the quadriceps muscles. The end. Not working yet? Here are some tips:

Get a wall behind you and then let your weight be fully supported by resting your butt against it. If the quads aren't relaxing it's usually because you're still ever-so-slightly bending your knees.

If the kneecaps are still not dropping, sit on the front edge of a chair, and keeping your heels on the ground, stretch your legs out in front of you. Let your legs fully straighten. See if you can relax your quads in this position.

Another reason your kneecaps won't drop could be because they're already down. To see if this is the case, tense your quads a few times and see if your kneecaps move upward. If they do, then congratulations, you're already practiced in releasing your quads.

Once you've mastered the quad release, it should be added to your other leg alignment points (feet straight, ankles ASIS width, neutral knee pits)—which isn't easy! You might find that you're tensing your quads in order to rotate your thigh; ideally this rotation should come from the deeper hip rotators and not require quad use.

▶ ILIACUS RELEASE

The iliacus is a muscle that runs between the pelvis and the femur and belongs to a group of muscles called the hip flexors. All hip flexors are forced to shorten to accommodate a sitting position. If you sit a lot, chances are this bugger has adapted. To see just how much resting tension you have between your pelvis and thigh:

Lie on your back (bolstering your ribs!) with your knees bent. Prop the inferior (closer to your legs) half of the pelvis up on a bolster, yoga block, or stack of towels, making sure to leave space under your waistband. Like a teeter-totter, your pelvis should tip toward your head, lowering your waistband toward the floor. If the pelvis doesn't rotate, then you've got a constant tug on your pelvis (and linea alba) that needs to be dealt with.

Don't work to rotate the pelvis; this defeats the point of "release." Just allow gravity to create this hip extension for you. Hang out here as long as you like, knowing that even if your pelvis doesn't budge, gravity is still creating the forces necessary to signal "lengthen!" to these muscles.

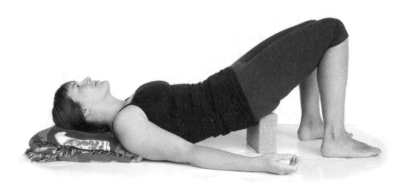

▶ PSOAS RELEASE

The psoas (pronounced *SO-az*) major is one doozie of a muscle, and you've got two of them.

Running down the length of your torso on each side of your spine, each psoas consists of a main muscle-body and eleven "fingers" that branch off, connecting to each vertebrae (and the discs in between) from your ribcage to your pelvis. Each of these muscles then goes on to connect to its respective thigh-bone, making a grand total of twenty-two attachments per pair of psoai (pronounced *SO-eye*). Also known as twenty-two places between which you can have too much tension and limited mobility. The psoai can thrust your ribs, pull on your discs, and move your lumbar spine out of whack. These muscles can also keep your legs positioned slightly out in front of you…all the time. Of course, thrusting your ribs and keeping your legs out in front of you can be caused by other muscles, resulting in a psoas adaptation that keeps you in that position, even if it wasn't the one that initiated the movement in the first place.

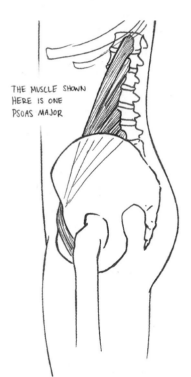

THE MUSCLE SHOWN HERE IS ONE PSOAS MAJOR

Wonky core geometry means wonky core function. Think of this psoas exercise as a sort of de-fragging of your core's computer. Clear out the tension-data that's slowing down the core muscles' ability to respond to the loads placed upon them.

Here's both an assessment and a way to get these puppies to let down your spine.

Start by sitting on the floor with legs extended. Relax the muscles of the thighs until the hamstrings rest on the ground. You might need to untuck your pelvis for this to happen.

Once your thighs are down, start to recline, stopping just before the hamstrings lift away from the ground. At this angle, bolster your head and shoulders, leaving space for the ribs to lower toward the floor. When your legs are straight with the hamstrings touching the floor, the height of the ribs from the floor is an indication of your habitual psoas tension (i.e., how much rib thrust is coming from the resting tension in your psoas). This bolstering technique is kind of like bolstering your ribs in the previous exercises, only this time you want space underneath the back of the ribs. Why? At some point you need to feel just how much you're actively thrusting your ribs. If you always bolster your entire upper body, there's never a chance to recognize and change the habit. In some exercises I have you bolster all the way, to complete the exercise. But the purpose of this exercise is **to learn to stop thrusting**, so I'm only having you bolster partway. (image top of next page)

Once you have identified and bolstered your head and shoulders, start relaxing the ribs to the floor. As with all the other "releasing" exercises, the point is not to get your ribcage to the floor by flexing your muscles, but to realize just how much you're tensing muscles and moving your own skeleton subconsciously. As you relax your psoas, your ribs will be able to move closer to the floor, so continuously adjusting the height or position of the bolster will be necessary as you improve.

Releasing your psoas can take anywhere from ten minutes to ten years, but coupling this exercise with constantly dropping your ribs throughout the day will result in a better overall tone to these muscles and a better geometry for your abdominal muscles.

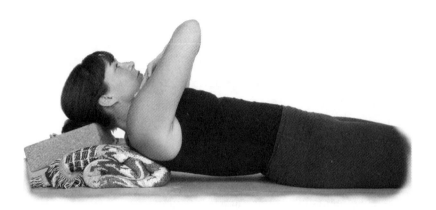

▸ RECTUS FEMORIS QUAD STRETCH

The psoas tends to take all the blame for restricted hip extension, when really the iliacus (a muscle between the pelvis and the thighbone) and the rectus femoris (RF, the only one of the four quadriceps muscles to run between the pelvis and the shin) are more involved with the hip joint. Many people try to stretch their quads, not realizing that one of the quads—the RF— passes over two joints (the hip and the knee). Thus it is easily and often blown past in "quad" exercises that don't fix both the pelvis and lower leg.

Do you want to meet a quad that's likely tugging your pelvis all the time? Here we go.

Starting on your belly, place a bolster—a rolled-up sleeping bag works great for this—under the front of your pelvis (put your ASIS, a.k.a. "hipbones," higher up on the roll) and let your pubic bone fall toward the floor. This will tilt your pelvis into place, making this next part of the exercise extremely effective.

To see how much tension is in this one quad, bend your knee to bring your ankle up to your hand, if you can reach it, without letting your pubic bone change position. You might find that your foot won't even reach your hand, so to stretch this one muscle, you might need a strap (or a belt or tie) to loop around your ankle so you can reach it with ease.

Note: Grab the lowest part of the shin and not the foot or toes. This will keep you from displacing the load to hyper-lax ankle ligaments instead of the rectus femoris.

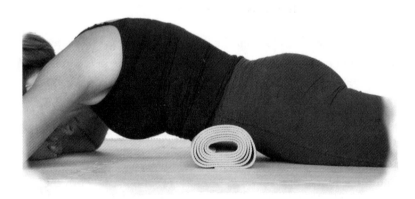

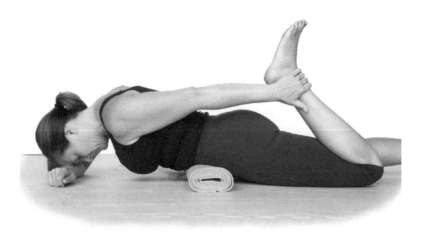

▶ THE LUNGE MAKEOVER

A lunge is a great way to measure the relationship between your pelvis and thigh. Start by sitting up on your knees, preferably on something soft, like carpet or a yoga mat. Step forward with your right leg and shift your weight forward to your front foot, lowering the pelvis toward the floor. Repeat other leg.

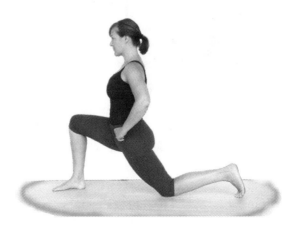

Okay, that was how most people do most lunges. I'm going to modify this a bit, though, so that it better demonstrates the actual relationship between the pelvis and thigh.

Start again, up on your knees, this time lining up your pelvis so that your pelvis is in neutral—keep the ASIS and pubic symphysis on a vertical plane, with the two top points above the bottom point so they all line up. Step forward with your right foot, and shift your weight forward toward the front foot as far as you can without your pelvis tilting.

If you need to, scoot your front foot forward, until you feel that your back leg can't extend any farther. Repeat other side.

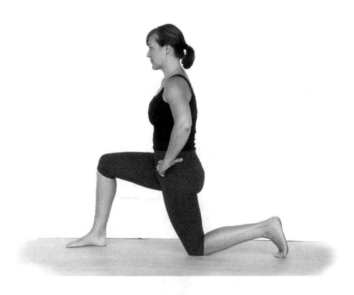

Maintaining the original position of your pelvis ensures that you isolate the muscles between the pelvis and thigh. In the first lunge it's likely that your pelvis tilted forward, thus straining the front of your abdomen. Because we want to stop straining our abdomen when we use our legs, we have to be mindful of how we execute all exercises—even ones that seem to be only for the legs.

▶ HIP SLIDE AND GLIDE

Stand in front of a chair with your feet a little wider than shoulder-width apart and bend forward, resting your hands on the seat of the chair. Relax the spine down toward the floor, without bending the arms. After you've relaxed the spine, back your hips up until they are behind your heels.

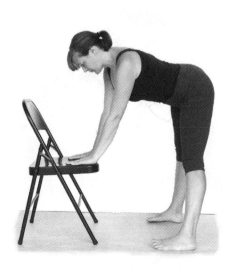

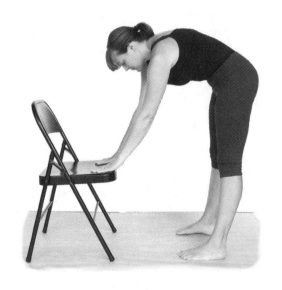

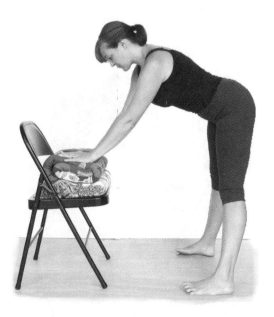

If your hamstrings are super tight and you find that, even after you relax your spine, your back is rounding up like a cat's, build up the height of the seat with books until your arms are holding your weight and your spine is relaxed and no longer rounded. (images on opposite page)

Shift your pelvis toward the right foot and then to the left. As you do this exercise, you'll be stretching the deeper muscles between the pelvis and femur.

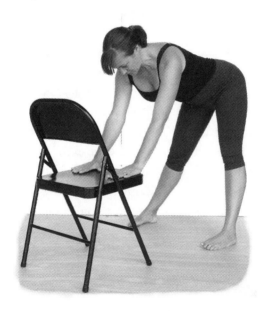

There are two ways to make this more challenging. The first is to rotate your thighs into neutral (as shown on page 68); this will bring your whole leg into a better alignment to load muscles that are affecting how your thigh and pelvis relate to each other when walking.

A second way to make this more challenging is to do the Slide and Glide with your butt against a wall. It's common to slightly move your pelvis forward, or hike it up on one side; both are very subtle cheats that reduce the impact of the exercise. Using a wall is like having a relentless personal trainer behind you.

I'll do this exercise as a sitting break (just get up, turn around, and *voila!*) a few times a day, for a couple of minutes each time. It's a great way to get a dynamic calf, hamstring, adductor, and deep hip stretch…all at the same time!

All of these exercises targeting the over-tight relationship between the pelvis and thighbones are necessary because of how much you have sat in the past. If you continue with the same habits that led your body to developing a DR, your healing and strengthening will be an extremely slow process. If you're sitting (i.e., practicing your hip-TENSING exercises) eight hours a day, and only doing one hour of corrective exercises each day, the math isn't in your favor. Don't panic! I've got how best to sit covered in chapter 8; I just wanted to remind you here that the need for correctives is coming from your smoking (I mean, sitting) habit.

ABDOMINAL EXERCISES

You're so excited, right? FINALLY, the stuff you've been waiting for. Well, guess what? Everything in this book is a core-strengthening exercise. The following are just a few isolated moves that will help you gauge not your core *strength*, necessarily, but your skills in monitoring, mobilizing, and stabilizing your ribs, pelvis, and spine to allow your core to participate.

▶ ROLL OVER, ROLL BACK

Rolling over from your back to your front was probably the first move you ever did as a baby. See how it goes for you now! Lie on your back with your legs straight and your arms stretched out over your head. Without lifting your head, arms, or legs, initiate a roll to your left and onto your stomach, and then once more in the same direction, so that you end up on your back. Then, repeat rolling to the opposite direction. Eventually your arms, legs, and head will move, but this exercise is to try to get you to initiate the work from the core muscles—just as you did it when you were a baby. It's easy to fling an arm or leg across the body and let gravity work on the limb and create the movement without using your core muscles—but that's not what we're after.

Repeat this process ten times.

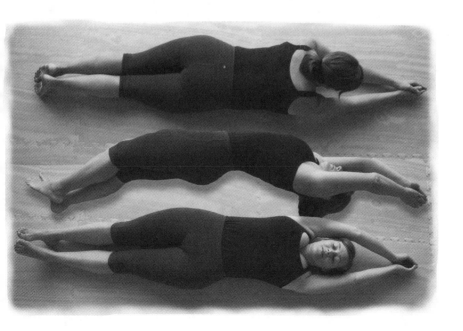

▸ THE ROCKING CHAIR

This exercise is fun. It can be a little challenging once I strip away all the cheats, but still, it's going to be fun. Especially once you get strong enough to *really* do it.

Are you excited?

I hope so.

Are your ribs down?

I hope so.

CORE CONFUSION

There are many exercises to train the transverse abdominis (TrA), but what I've noticed is, when people demonstrate those exercises for me, all they're doing is tucking the pelvis under while they "activate their transverse." Here's the thing: the TrA does not have the attachments to move the pelvis, so if drawing in your belly button is moving your pelvis, you might be suffering from some core confusion.

Try this: **In front of a mirror**, climb down onto your hands and knees. Assume a neutral-pelvis, neutral-ribcage position, and relax your belly. Without holding your breath (keep breathing, won't you please?), pull your belly button up toward your spine, watching in the mirror the entire time. Your pelvis should not budge at all! If your pelvis tucked—see page 111 for a picture—then go back and try it again, trying to find a different way to lift your abdominal wall up. Keep trying until you can pull the belly button in, without holding your breath and without tucking the pelvis. This isn't an exercise to do often, but rather a test to break up any inappropriate relationships between abdominal engagement and pelvis tucking you've established in your mind.

Start by lying on your back, with your knees in toward your chest. Wrap your arms underneath your shins so that you're holding your thighs close to your body, and then grab each arm's wrist or elbow to keep your legs in place. Maintaining your grip will make sure your legs will not be generating momentum for you, and that your hip flexors won't be trying to do the work.

Lift your head and shoulders off the ground, making your body the shape of a rocking chair. Without straining (and I can't stress "without straining" enough; if you're grunting and struggling with this exercise, come back to it after you've been doing the others for some time), rock your body back and forth between the bottom of your ribs and just below your waistband. Do not go any higher or lower than these markers.

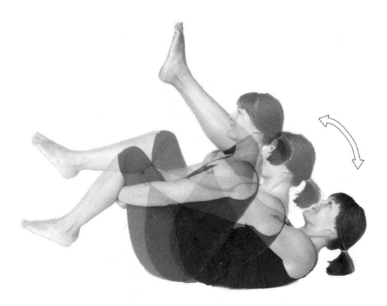

Ideally, the area between your ribs and pelvis should flex (curve) with ease, but when you've been a long-time thruster, as so many of us are, the vertebrae in that part of your spine have been displaced in a way that prevents them from flexing easily. This exercise creates loads that can gently move these vertebrae back "home" as well as restore appropriate mobility. If your floor is especially hard, fold a towel a couple of times to create a softer surface for this area of your spine.

If you're unable to move at all—if that area of the body won't curve and just stays a flat line—go back and work on the Click-Clack (page 99) for a few more weeks, then check back to see if this one is getting any easier for you!

▶ ROCKING CHAIR 360

Once you've mastered a core-driven rocking chair, start turning yourself around in small increments with every rock until you've spun yourself around 360 degrees. Then do the same thing in the opposite direction. You should look graceful while doing this exercise. Just kidding. You'll probably make some super-gross faces while you do it, but it's also very fun and challenging. If you notice yourself straining—grunting and gasping and throwing your body forward and back—**you're not ready for this exercise yet**. You should be able to breathe easily throughout—a sign that you're not messing with your pressures (and straining your linea alba and/or pelvic floor) while doing this exercise.

All of the exercises in the last two chapters have been priming your body to move more. But moving more is only really moving more if more of you moves when you exercise. You've probably gathered by now that parts of your body have been clumped together, and this clumpy motion tends to hinge on the linea alba. These smaller micronutrient-type moves will change the loads created when you go out and move more...move bigger. Which is what's coming up next.

CRUNCH CONTRAINDICATIONS

Despite great advances in our understanding of core conditioning, abdominal "crunch" exercises are still the go-to ab workout for most people. While I have no problem with any type of human movement, the increase in intra-abdominal pressure created by the crunch motion (and exacerbated by many repetitions of it) can be problematic if you're trying to repair an issue created, in part, by too much intra-abdominal pressure. The same goes for planks and any sort of isometric exercise you strain to maintain (as opposed to move through).

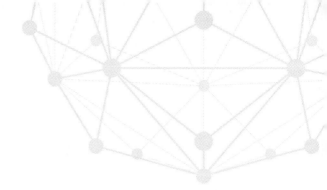

BIG MOVES

CHAPTER 8

If there's one message I'd like to get across to you it's this: Your core is not weak because you didn't do enough ab exercises or because you did the wrong ab exercises. Your core muscles are weak because they have been used very little—both in terms of frequency and variability. The tissues of your core are behaving exactly as a biomechanist would expect given the information about how you have moved over a lifetime.

SITTING TIME

I'm starting this Big Moves section with "sitting" because of the great frequency with which you sit. You sit BIG time. Which is understandable. We live in a chair-based culture. Our education and employment systems require that we sit, our family time is often spent sitting around a table to share food or on a couch to share entertainment, and our spiritual practices typically require long bouts of stillness. When it comes to core strength, the amount of time we sit has limited the function of the abdominal muscles much more than a lack of abdominal exercise has, and so we absolutely have to discuss sitting in a book about waning core function.

TAKE THE "HOW MUCH DO I SIT?" QUIZ:

All answers must be in minutes and should relate to an average day.
- Commute time to and from work: _____
- Commute time for kids to after-school activities: _____
- Riding a bike: _____
- Sitting at work: _____
- Sitting eating breakfast, lunch, and dinner: _____
- Watching TV/movies (30–60 minutes per show):_____
- Using the Internet or computer (not at work): _____
- Other sitting time (reading, playing instruments, sewing, knitting, toilet, building models, etc.): _____
- Total minutes sitting (add all numbers above): _____
- Calculate your sleep time: 420 minutes (7 hours) is the average amount of time most people sleep a day, but you can adjust this number up or down depending if you sleep, read, or laze in bed less or more.
- Write your "bedtime" minutes here: _____
- Subtract the above number from 1440 (the total number of minutes in a day):
- 1440 - bedtime minutes = Amount of daily available "moving" time.
- 1440 – _____ = _____

This final value is the amount of waking time you have in a day; a period of time where you could be (and would be) moving through numerous body positions and loads if movement were still necessary for survival.

If you divide your total minutes sitting by your number of daily moving minutes, and multiply by 100, you will have the percentage of each day you spend in almost the exact same position.

You spend _____ % of every day sitting and not using your core muscles dynamically (i.e., in a way that would utilize them in many different directions, with many different loads, and result in well-balanced muscle mass and yield).

With the numbers right there in your hand, you can begin to see the magnitude of the problem. Don't freak out. I have a three-step plan that will allow you to make big progress: sit better, sit differently, sit less.

SIT BETTER

I'm fully expecting you to sit less in the future, but before you figure out how to make small changes in your sitting habits here and there, you can learn to sit better. Sitting better simply means sitting in a way that uses more muscle actively. When you sit, the problem is not only that your entire body is inactive (i.e., you're sedentary); your body is likely leaning into the furniture you are using. Slouching into a chair or even into your own spine is a way for your body to conserve energy, but because we sit so much and because there are almost no movements required of our body in a modern, technology-based society, we end up with failing tissues in the midsection. Slouching or using furniture is fine every now and then, but because "doing nothing" with our abdominal muscles makes up almost the entire mechanical experience of the core, we get a core that performs "not much"—because that's what we've done with it.

▸ SIT NEAR THE FRONT OF YOUR CHAIR

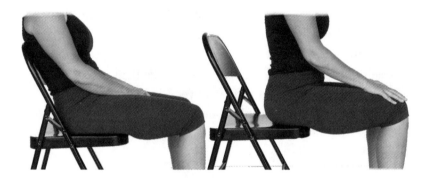

An easy "sitting makeover" is to scoot your body toward the front of your chair so you are unable to use the spinal support. Don't worry, you come with your own spinal support. We call them core muscles. See? That chair was robbing you of a chance to work your body, making it so that after you were done sitting for work, you had to go work out. Sitting near the front edge of your chair also makes it easier for you to maintain a neutral pelvis (see next point), while simultaneously making it more difficult for you to lean against the back of it.

▶ UNTUCK YOUR PELVIS

Okay, even though you're away from the backrest of a chair, your body is clever; eventually you'll start to slump and round your spine, creating a similar "body resting" effect. Again, this slump is totally natural ("bad posture" is a cultural idea), but, because the amount of time you spend sitting is *un*natural, you're going to have to adjust yourself out of this slump a lot.

As you sit on the edge of your chair, roll your pelvis forward as though it's a bowl of soup you're trying to pour out the front, until your ASIS and pubic symphysis are in vertical alignment (a.k.a. "neutral pelvis"). To make this pelvic motion bigger (i.e., easier to feel), sit on a rolled towel. The height of the towel will create an exaggerated motion that you can use to get a feel for the move, or to play with tucking and untucking as an "undercover exercise" you can do while sitting at work.

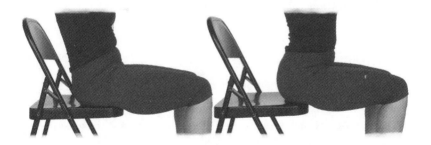

▶ DE-HUMP YOUR UPPER BACK

Keeping your ribs down and starting with your chin on your chest, work to bring your head and eyes level to the horizon. If you only bring your head up, your chin will jut forward, moving only the uppermost vertebrae in your neck. As you can imagine, the constant impingement of the skull and the neck's vertebrae isn't great for those tissues, nor does it help the upper back that's still sitting there rounded over.

So, arrange your sternum and lower your chin to your chest again. This time, without lifting the chin *or* moving the ribcage, bring your eyes up to the horizon by moving the vertebrae in the upper back. Think of sliding the back of your head to the wall behind you, while lifting the crown of the head up to the ceiling. The movement here will be small at first, but you should, maybe for the first time, feel work in the muscles that move the upper curved part of your spine.

Every time you take a seat, scoot away from any back support it's trying to foist on you, adjust your pelvis, arrange your middle back (drop your ribs), and lift your head (not your chin) to the ceiling. These constant adjustments will set the stage for better core activation *while you're just sitting there.*

SIT DIFFERENTLY

Sitting is not sitting is not sitting. Many of the corrective exercises we do to change the tension between the muscles of the legs and pelvis can be accomplished while you're sitting—or rather, while you're *stationary.* YES, you can be stationary and still work on exercises to improve your core function. All you have to do is sit differently.

Consider your most common chair- or couch-sitting postures, and you'll find that they're almost all exactly the same. It's this sameness that allows the muscles to tense and the loads to the linea alba to stay constant.

What you can do, right now while you're reading this book, is to sit cross-legged on a chair; sit on a bolster or pillow and spread your legs in a wide V; sit directly on the floor; sit on your knees. It's okay if you're not able to stay in any one position for long or if you need to add pillows under your hips to make this new way of sitting comfortable. It only matters that you change something about the geometry in your hips. Oh, and also that you drop your ribs.

Are you dropping your ribs? Good. Just checking. Again.

SIT LESS

I've worked with you on sitting, you can't deny it. You've sat better, and you've sat differently. At some point, though, you're going to have to swap some of your sitting time for non-sitting time. Yup, you're going to have to sit less.

▸ IDEAS TO REDUCE SITTING TIME

- Look for times you can reduce the amount of unnecessary (i.e., non-work) time you spend in a chair.

- Consider eating some meals standing at the counter.

- Lie on the floor or do stretches while you watch TV.

- Kneel while you fold laundry instead of sitting on the bed.

- If you take public transit, consider standing for at least some of the journey.

- Walk instead of driving, or drive partway, and walk the rest.

- Swap sitting on the toilet for squatting with a squat platform. Bonus: Straining during bathrooming can increase intra-abdominal pressure; a Squatty Potty can improve how you "go."

These changes might seem small, but they are mighty, and the less time you spend sitting, the more effective the corrective movements you do will be!

STANDING (DYNAMIC) WORKSTATION

For those of you doing a lot of office and computer work, begin to transition to a standing workstation. Physiologically, your body is probably not ready for you to stand for a full workday, but that's okay. In fact, it's better to mix up your working postures—to create a dynamic workstation, if you will.

Try standing up to work for 10 percent of your computer time at first—fifty minutes of an eight-hour day. This doesn't have to be all at once—in fact, it will be more beneficial to spread those fifty minutes out over the rest of your work time, changing between standing and sitting fairly frequently.

Another great way to sit less is to be moving more. The following is a list of moving activities that not only reduce your sitting time, they increase the amount (in terms of minutes) and the way (in terms of which muscles and how much) you use your core.

WALKING

In a less convenient society, we'd all be walking three to five miles most days, along with a semi-regular long-distance walk of eight to ten miles. Don't worry, you can work up to that kind of mileage slowly. Also, you don't have to do all your walking at once; it's just as beneficial to your core muscles, if not more, to

SUCCESS TIP: FIND A WALKING BUDDY

I can't tell you how much a walking buddy will improve your success at logging your daily miles. Here is what I suggest: Go to Facebook right now and post this: "Looking for an early morning walking buddy (or group of buddies!) to meet me three to five days a week, to do three to five miles. If you're not interested but have friends who might be and live in my area, will you please share? Thanks!"

This is how I found my walking buddy, and I'm happy to say we're still walking most days a week over a year later!

spread it out over the day, breaking up long bouts of stillness.

Keeping in mind that I have two young children (three and four years at the time of writing this book) and a very busy work schedule, my favorite way to get my walking in is to get up early, before the rest of my family, and meet a friend for a long walk while the sun comes up. I then take a couple of slow, exploring walks during the day with my children, and sometimes, weather permitting, another one after they go to sleep. We walk to the post office, to the grocery store, to forest school. We've made hiking our family pastime, allowing us to further increase our movement while spending time learning, laughing, and being together on weekends and holidays.

I also look to my schedule to see where I can blend errands and walking to get a ten- or fifteen-minute walk here or there. Consider your planner. Can you take work phone calls and meetings outside for a stroll? Could you walk to the grocery store for a few items? How about managing one half-hour or hour-long walk in the morning, or at lunchtime? Every step is of benefit to your core and therefore to your whole body.

HANGING

Let's face it, our arms rarely do more than text or type. And because texting and typing use very little of your core muscles, the large force productions your core muscles are capable of creating never happen.

We think of diastasis recti as an issue local to the abdomen, probably because we don't like the way our stomach looks when we have a DR. But for the sake of seeing the larger picture, in order to have a strong-in-many-ways core, you have to use your abdominals in many ways, throughout a day and over a lifetime. This is what gives you an amount of strength and resting tone capable of keeping your innards in place.

As I mentioned earlier, your core muscles connect your lower body to your upper, so a lifetime of barely using your arms will always leave a large portion of your abdominal strength under-utilized. This is the section where we change all of that.

Hanging, swinging, and carrying stuff in your arms are totally natural things to do. Only, we no longer live in nature, and so we must begin by gently introducing these loads to our body. The good news: you've already been progressing toward these skills by improving your shoulder and rib mobility. **If you have a connective tissue issue as mentioned on page 44, this is a reminder to keep your feet on the ground at all times and only progress when you can execute and exercise without losing the alignment points I've mentioned for your safety.**

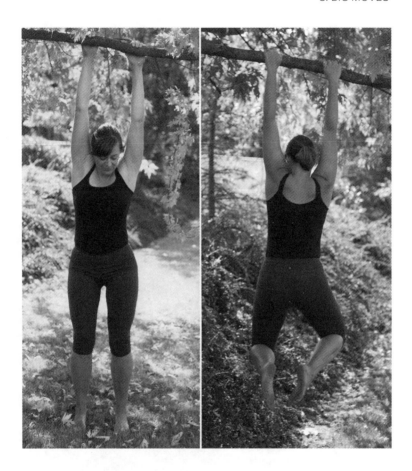

Your upper-body and core training starts with very low loads. To do this, you'll need to find a bar or branch that allows you to keep your feet on the ground. Holding on with both arms, slowly bend your knees, dropping the weight of your body away from your hands. **Watch to make sure your elbows don't straighten beyond 180°. If they do, put a small bend in your elbows and work to maintain it.** This will protect the ligaments in your elbows. (image top left)

Once you can stabilize your elbows, find a bar that allows you to hang with your feet off the ground. Check your shoulder blades; are they up at your ears? See if you can **bring them down toward your waistband**, and…you guessed it…see if you can keep your ribs down. When you're hanging with your shoulders and ribs down and you're breathing, you should feel the muscles in your midsection working. (previous page, right image)

SWINGING

Once you've mastered the hang, see if you can get your body swinging forward and back. Although you're always the same weight, this type of movement creates a larger load, and it's a nice way to increase the work to your abdominals (and everything else). See if you can work up to ten swings. Remember, **if you're not able to keep your elbows from over-extending and your shoulders down, then back up a step** and practice the static hang more often.

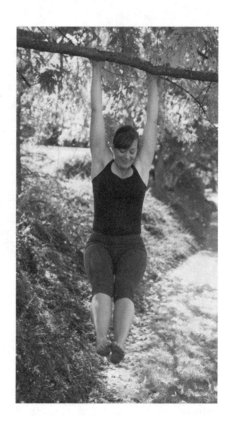

Another type of swinging, which will better prepare you for one-armed hanging and swinging, is a side-to-side swing.

You'll be using your waist muscles to get your legs swinging right to left, like a pendulum. Just as in the other hangs and swings, keep the shoulders and the ribs down to better utilize the muscles in your trunk.

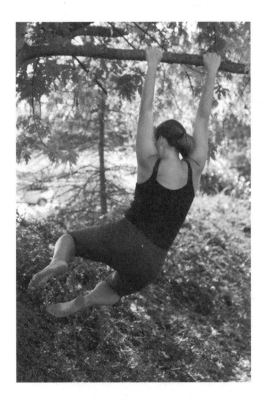

THE MONKEY BARS

Swinging down the monkey bars is similar to walking; it's essentially a one-armed hang, followed by another, and another. It takes time to go from being able to do a double-armed hang to a single one as it's twice the work, so only progress as your body indicates better strength. **You can gauge this by your ability to stabilize your elbows.**

TALK ABOUT WHOLE BODY!

Hanging doesn't only benefit your core muscles; it's great for developing strong arms and shoulders. And there's something even larger at play. A 2015 study (find it under Leong in the reference section) showed that grip strength was a stronger predictor of all-cause and cardiovascular mortality than systolic blood pressure. When we see a headline touting the benefits of "grip strength," especially one citing a study like this, we might feel like running out and training with a series of grip-strength exercises to reap the protective effects. However, grip-strength exercises are probably not what these (100,000+) study participants were doing. It's more likely that they were using their shoulders, arms, and hands more throughout the day, for exercise, work, or hobbies.

If you'd like to improve your grip strength and core and upper-body strength, do it all at once, via whole-body movement macronutrients that challenge your parts with the weights of your body—like these exercises in the hanging, swinging, and carrying section!

CARRYING
....

When you first have a DR, carrying stuff can cause pain in your back. However, oftentimes life presents us with the need to carry things, like our kids or groceries. The fact of the matter is, if you carried things more often, your body would be better conditioned to deal with the ever-changing loads created by carrying things of different sizes and weights. Instead of waiting to carry something in an emergency, train for it, keeping in mind that your core will respond best to a constant variance in loads. Here are my steps to better carrying technique:

Fix your base. The base of carrying is everything your arms attach to. Line up your feet and knees, stack your pelvis, drop your ribs, and then assume the load.

Constantly shift how you carry. You don't need to center your load all of the time. The "centering" is more an average of loads over the day. If you're carrying a baby, for example, carry a while on your right and a while on your left side. A while on your back, and a while on your front. The same goes for carrying a backpack or purse. Do you always carry it in the same way? Switch arms, test out your new grip strength and your core in a unique way. Think of your core muscles as a tube capable of a hundred different ways of working as a unit. In order to elicit a broad distribution of strength, your job is to constantly change things up. Variety is the spice of life and a key to a well-adapted structure.

Carry often. Ditch the stroller and carry your kid in your arms, even if it's only for a short period of time. Walk to the grocery store and carry that gallon of milk in your hands instead of in a bag. Stack your own wood in the winter (or find some other chore and reclaim the movement you've outsourced). Our lives

MOVE

are full of "conveniences" that save us time, but sap our strength. Carrying stuff is more work, but that's why you bought a book with exercises in it, right?

▸ GET DOWN, GET UP

You're going to be excited about this exercise because you get to sit for part of it. Here's how to do it.

- Go sit on the floor.
- Get back up again.
- Go sit on the floor in a different way.
- Get back up again.
- Repeat until you've sat down and gotten up ten times.

I've said it before, and I'll say it again: The best piece of exercise equipment you're not using is your floor. There is a distance there—between the seat of your favorite chair and the ground—that is almost never traversed by your knees and hips. It takes a lot of work to lower down and lift up your body weight, and in a less furniture-filled setting, you'd be doing this motion twenty times a day. You might not think of getting up and down off the floor as core work, but that's probably because you're using your hands a lot. As you get used to getting up and down, try using your hands less. Less pushing your hands into the floor, less pushing your hands on your thighs—and more core and hip muscle use.

▸ THE SIT AND SHIFT

This is perhaps the most challenging exercise in this section, and my favorite.

Start by sitting with your legs tucked underneath you, with your knees bent and your feet under your bottom. (This might not be a super comfortable way to sit at first, in which case you need to pause the exercise here, and just sit like this frequently until it is more comfortable. Yes, sitting with your legs tucked underneath you can be an exercise if you're not used to doing it!)

Then lower your right hip to the right, until it is resting on the ground.

SUCCESS TIP: AT A PLAYGROUND? DON'T JUST SIT THERE!

If you have children there's a good chance that you find yourself someplace "for the kids" and just sit there, waiting until you're free later on to work out. Guess what? You can be accomplishing big and small movement tasks while still being there for your family. Waiting for practice to be over? Walk laps around the field or do some of the stretches in this book. Find yourself at a park or playground? I make it a rule NEVER to sit down at a playground. Instead, I challenge my core with as many hangs and monkey-bar crossings as I can do before my hands give out. While I'm letting my hands rest from that, I'll climb the play structure, creating small challenges like not using my hands for balance or scaling the outside of the structure. In fact, quite often I'll invite my adult friends to work out at the park and, of course, encourage them to bring their kids!

See if you can somehow coordinate one of your daily walks to bring you to a place with bars or trees for some hanging and swinging practice!

If your waist is very tight, **bolster this exercise by placing a folded bath towel just to the right and left sides of your hips,** in which case you only have to lower your right hip to the height of the towel.

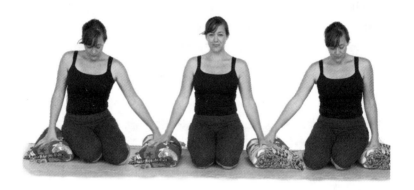

Sit here for a moment, and then, using the muscles in your waist, lower body, and a little momentum, shift your hips to the left. Try to keep your torso upright and your ribs down (of course!), as you shift from side to side. You don't need to do this quickly; rather, you're seeing how well you can change the position of your body utilizing the muscles of the waist. This shifting is a complex motion. It's not a contrived "oblique exercise" but rather a natural movement that involves your entire torso in a dynamic and functional way. As you improve, work to reduce your bolstering and your momentum.

MYOFASCIA: GET ON THE BALL

Around, between, and through all of your parts winds a tissue called fascia. This connective tissue's role in structure and movement has been essentially ignored in anatomy throughout history. Recently fascia has become better understood and is being added back into anatomical models, especially when it comes to holistic functions like movement and stability. With a better understanding of fascia have come modalities specific to improving this tissue's function, and thus overall movement and mobility. Many of these treatments require a device of some type, shaped specifically to get in between your smaller parts—to create motion where none has occurred in some time.

In the case of the abdomen, I've found moving the body around and over balls and rollers of various sizes, textures, and densities creates subtle movements and loads that are difficult to replicate in the modern world. When done in conjunction with moving better and moving more, these additional movements can improve your outcomes.

A series of moves (big to small) I use to mobilize the waist:

• Big Ball: Draping over an exercise ball
Keeping your feet on the floor, scissor your legs wide so that the top leg is in back and the bottom leg is in front of you. Arc your body over the ball, without rolling your torso and pelvis forward or back.
(image top of next page)

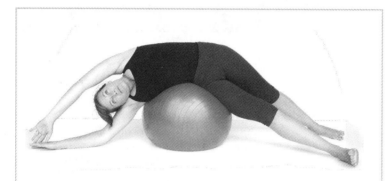

• Medium Ball: Ball in the guts

Okay, don't really put this ball in your guts. In fact, you're going to stay off of your midline and linea alba altogether and instead stick to the muscles just outside the lineae semilunaris. Lie on your abdomen, placing the medium ball (modeling Yoga Tune Up®'s Coregeous® ball here) just to the right of the semilunaris. Allow your body to relax over the ball. As you reduce any bracing tension in your obliques, the ball will sort of sink into your muscle. Move your body toward your head, and toward your feet, "vacuuming" over this entire half of your waist. Give yourself five to ten minutes, looking for spots that aren't relaxing well. Repeat on the other side.

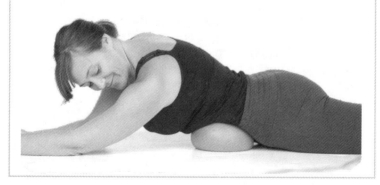

• **Small Ball**

RIB THRUSTERS, HEAR THIS. Your muscles, especially those on your back, between your pelvis and waist (the quadratus lumborum) have to stiffen to keep that rib thrust going. Which means that even if you try to drop your ribs, muscles adapted to "ribs up" can be working against you (and gravity, for that matter, so don't take it personally). I'm a fan of lying on my back, knees bent, and pinning a small ball (tennis ball or one designed specifically for this purpose) between the right side of my waist—just above the pelvis— and the ground. Bringing the right knee into the chest, I'll rock my body right and left to massage my waist muscles with the ball. Then, I'll repeat the other side.

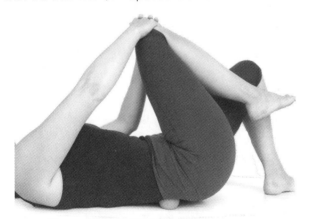

There are many different exercises you can do with the ball that can facilitate your progress. Self-fascial therapy programs typically require the purchase of specific products and often address the entire body. For this reason (the additional products, not because fascia is less important), I've included fascia as a sidebar and made a list of books, products, and programs that can assist your progress towards a well-functioning core in Appendix 1.

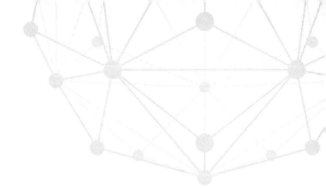

DROP YOUR RIBS

CHAPTER 9

D rop your ribs. That is all. I just wanted to put this here in case you were skimming the book and didn't read anything but the first line of the chapter. Just drop them. The end.

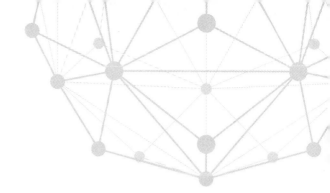

CONCLUSION: CHANGE

If I had titled this book *Diastasis Recti: The Whole LIFE Solution to Abdominal Weakness and Separation,* I probably would have scared many people away from reading it, but since you've made it this far, hear me out.

You've learned that for a stronger, more functional abdomen, you can change the shoes you wear, the clothes you wear, how you sit, how much you sit, how you stand, how you exercise, and how you move. (Okay, so changing your shoes might not seem like changing your LIFE, but maybe that's because you haven't started looking for totally flat shoes yet. They're not that easy to find—although the situation is improving.)

The benefit to changing these small things in your day-to-day life is that you'll be changing how you feel, how you look, and how you function—for the better.

There's nothing I'd like more than to give you Four Exercises That Will Flatten Your Abs or The Only 8 Minutes of Exercise You'll Ever Need, but if my years spent studying human movement have taught me anything, it is that you are a single body fashioned out of trillions of smaller bodies that are responding to all of your all-day behaviors. Changing your body's environment, then, is quite possibly the key to achieving the level of health you want—more so than any exercises you can do within the same environment that led your body to the state it is currently in. If the physical outcome of your body isn't working for your life, then it's the life that has to change to get your body working.

Don't worry about perfection; there are so many variables you can work with, so many entryways to feeling better. Just pick one thing—any one thing[1]—and begin. You can do it. I know you can.

---

1. Make sure you pick dropping your ribs.

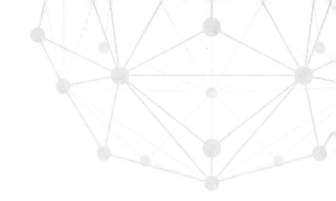

THE PROGRAM

BODY NEUTRAL

▸ **FEET PELVIS-WIDTH APART**

• Line up the middle of the front of your ankles with the bony prominences at the front of your pelvis (your ASIS).

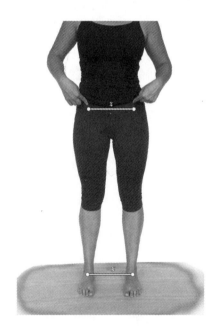

▶ BACK YOUR HIPS UP

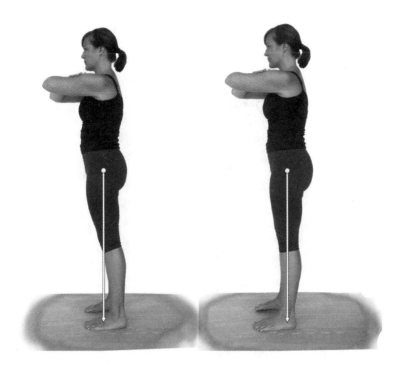

• Move your hips back so that they're directly over the knees and ankles. A plumb line should pick up the center of the hip joint, the midpoint of the knee, and the quarter-sized ankle bone over the heel.

▸ NEUTRAL FEMURS

- Point your feet straight ahead, so that the lateral malleoli (the outer quarter-sized ankle bones) are in line with the bony prominence just behind the pinkie toes.

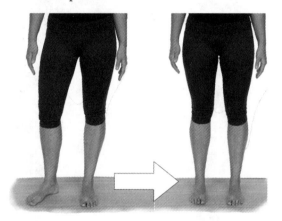

- Standing with a mirror behind you, turn your thighbones (usually away from each other) until the four lines down the back of both knees line up like this:

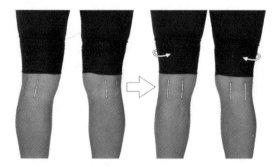

- You do not need to keep the instep of the foot down as you rotate your thighs to neutral.

▸ NEUTRAL PELVIS

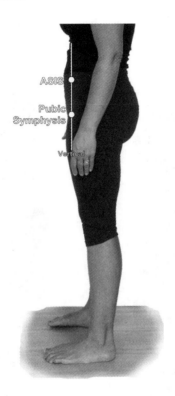

- Arrange the ASIS and the pubic symphysis vertically.
- Straining to attain a neutral pelvis is really an indication that you need to do your correctives more often as well as decrease any behaviors that are training your body away from the positioning you desire.

▶ DROP YOUR RIBS

• Shift your ribcage down and back until the bottom front ribs are aligned vertically with the ASIS and the pubic symphysis.

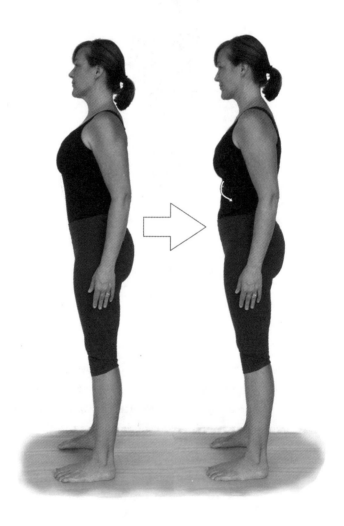

▸ RELEASE YOUR DIAPHRAGM

• Place your hands on your upper abdomen and allow your entire belly to relax, paying special attention to the sensation of your diaphragm releasing.

• You will probably feel your abdominal contents moving outward, both sensing the motion and feeling it with your hands.

• Once you feel you've released your diaphragm, try again—chances are you are holding residual tension there.

• Throughout the day, remind yourself to relax your diaphragm.

• For a more advanced version of the diaphragm release, relax your belly to the floor while on your hands and knees.

SMALL MOBILIZING EXERCISES

▸ FLOOR ANGELS

• Recline on a bolster or stacked pillows so that your ribcage can lower toward the floor.

• Reach your arms out to the side, keeping the palms facing up and the elbows lifting up toward the ceiling.

• Try to get the backs of your hands to the floor, keeping your elbows slightly bent.

• Once your chest can handle this stretch, slowly move your arms toward your head, only going as far as you can keeping your thumbs on the floor while trying to lift the elbows away from the floor.

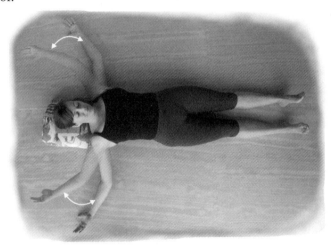

• Keep your ribs down and stable.

• Make a "snow angel" motion ten times, moving slowly and making sure to not go any higher than you can with your ribs down.

▶ WINDMILL STRETCH

• Starting on your back, bring your right knee up toward your chest and then roll your entire body to the left—don't spinal twist, but roll—until your right knee rests on the ground.
• Make sure your ribs are not thrusting.
• Reach your right hand, arm, and shoulder blade up toward the ceiling and away from the spine.
• Slowly drop your arm to the right as far as you can without thrusting your ribcage (it's okay if it doesn't go to the floor) until you find the boundary of your tension.
• Once there, imagine your arm is on the face of a clock. Keeping your palm facing the ceiling, slowly move your arm between twelve and six o'clock and then back up again.

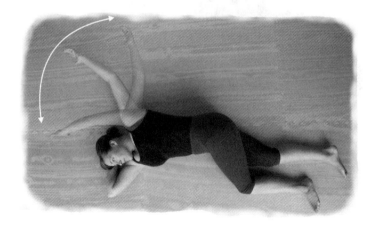

• Do this ten to fifteen times, continuously reaching your elbow away from your torso and checking that you're not thrusting your ribs!
• Repeat on the other side.

▶ DOORWAY WALKTHROUGH

• Every time you walk through a doorway, reach your arms up until you can touch the wall above it, and then drop your ribs back to neutral.

• Keeping the arms straight, step forward to increase the stretch, but really focus on dropping your ribs.

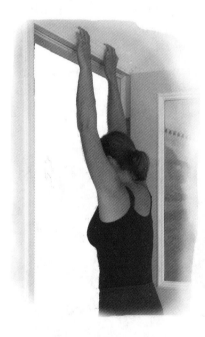

• Try a few with your elbows pointing straight ahead and see how movements of the shoulder change the load and the tendency to compensate with the ribs.

• If you can, loop your fingers around an edge and lower your weight towards the floor, doing the bulk of the work with your legs but a smidge of work with your arms.

• If you find yourself unable to reach the top of a doorway, you can do a single-armed version of this exercise, doing one arm at a time, one on the right and then left side of a doorway.

SMALL STRENGTHENING EXERCISES

▶ LOG PULLOVER

- Lie on your back with your legs extended on the floor. Grip the ends of a log and squeeze your elbows toward each other (tight shoulders may make them want to poke out to the right and left).
- Keeping the ribs down, lower the log overhead, only going as far as you can without letting the ribs lift up toward the ceiling, then bring the log back up to the starting position. Repeat fifteen to twenty times.

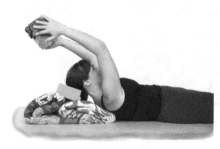

- When you first begin this exercise, you'll likely need to keep your ribs bolstered in order for them to stay neutral to the pelvis.
- As your shoulders become more mobile, you can remove the bolstering and use this same exercise as an abdominal strengthener.

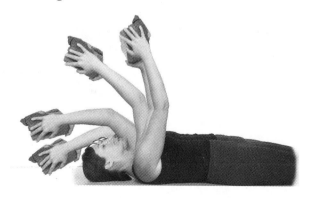

▸ ACTIVATE YOUR INTERCOSTALS

• Seated or standing, tie a resistance band or pair of tights firmly around your torso just beneath your chest muscles or breasts (at the height of a bra strap or heart rate monitor).

• Make sure you've dropped your ribs.

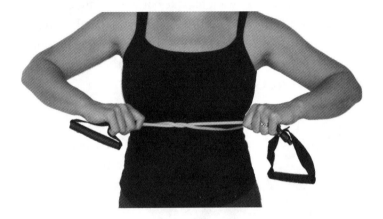

• Inhale deeply, expanding the ribcage into the band until you feel the resistance from the elastic pushing on your ribs.

• If you don't feel it at the end of your inhale, re-tie the band and try it again.

• Exhale, being aware of how your ribcage can pull away from the ring of elastic and closer to an imaginary vertical pole running up through the center of your body.

• Repeat, using each exhale to pull the ribs in and downward.

• Once you've got the motor skill, you can do this exercise without the tactile assistance of the band.

FREE UP YOUR WAIST

▸ FLOOR CRESCENT

• Lying on your back, interlace your fingers and reach your arms overhead until your wrists touch the ground.

• Bolster your upper body until your ribs are down.

• Once your ribs are down, walk your arms and legs to the right as far as possible, keeping all four limbs on the floor.

• If your shoulders are tight, keeping the arms on the ground might cause the ribs to pop up. If this happens, modify by allowing the arms to come up as necessary.

• To start to work at tight waist/hip muscles, cross your left ankle over your right to increase the stretch.

• You can also practice your intercostal activation breathing while holding this stretch for a minute or so.

• Repeat on the other side.

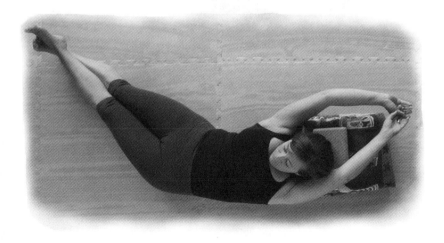

▶ SEATED SPINAL TWIST

- Sit in a chair with a neutral pelvis and your ribs down.
- Without jutting your ribs or tucking or untucking your pelvis, turn to the right and to the left without straining.
- Move to the edge of your range of motion, taking care that you're not slightly moving out of alignment to go farther.
- Once you've done this a few times, hold to one side, practicing the active intercostal exhale for 5 breaths.
- Then twist back and forth a few times and hold the twist to the other side (ribs down), doing the active intercostal exhale again, for 5 breaths.
- Complete the circuit with a few twists back and forth.

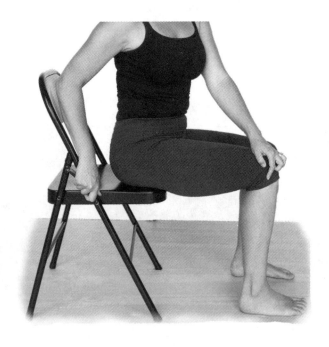

▸ BOLSTERED SPINAL TWIST

• Lying on your back, bolster your upper body until your ribs are down.

• Once you're bolstered, scoot your pelvis an inch or two to the right, then bring the right knee up so that it stacks over your hip, and rotate your pelvis to lower that knee to the opposite side of your body, stopping as soon as your ribs start to leave the ground.

• Twist only as far as you can without taking the ribs with you—no forcing it.

• If you find that your pelvis barely moves and your knee is nowhere near the floor, stack pillows so that the knee crossing over can rest on them. This will reduce the load to the spine and keep these muscles from tensing unnecessarily.

• Repeat on the other side.

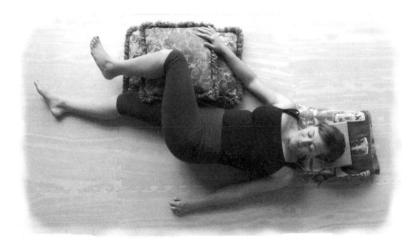

▸ RIB SLIDE ON THE WALL

• Stand against a wall with your feet spread a bit wider than pelvis width, and get yourself lined up so that, while your feet remain a few inches from the wall, your bottom and your bra strap (or bro strap) are on the wall, and your ribs are D-O-W-N.

• Slide your ribs to the right and left, creating a horizontal movement that requires the muscles between the ribs and pelvis to loosen up.

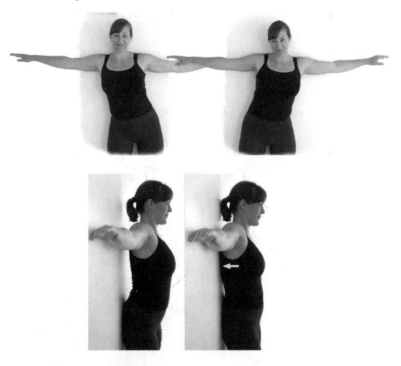

• Shoulders and ribcage stay level as they move to the right and left of your pelvis.

• Eventually you won't need a wall to do this exercise.

▶ CLICK-CLACK

- Start by sitting on the floor on a folded towel, which will create a bolster that makes the motion easier to do at first.

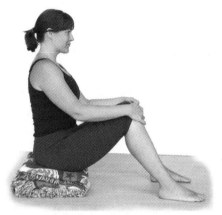

- See if you can tuck and untuck your pelvis, doing this however you can.
- Once you have some mobility, bend your knees until your feet are flat on the ground.
- Holding onto your shins just below the knee, lean back until your arms are straight, and keep your ribs down. (cont'd next page)

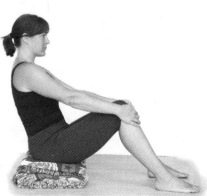

▸ CLICK-CLACK CONT'D

• Keep your body in this position (especially the straight arms and ribs down and feet down) throughout the exercise. (image on previous page)

• Without changing your arm length, tilt your pelvis forward and back, noticing the tendency to want to lift the chest and tense the muscles in your back. At first, your only job is to keep the arms straight and ribs down while articulating only your pelvis.

• Once this is easy for you, begin to steer the motion of your pelvis *with your feet*.

• Keeping the feet in place (i.e., they're not going to go anywhere), fire all the muscles you would if you wanted your feet to slide away from you—but don't let them.

• Firing those muscles while holding your feet in place will force the upper part of your pelvis behind you, rolling over your ischial tuberosities (sitting bones) and tucking your pelvis.

• To get your pelvis to tilt forward, do the opposite foot work: try to draw your feet closer to you without letting them move and you'll rotate the top of your pelvis forward, creating an anterior (forward) tilt.

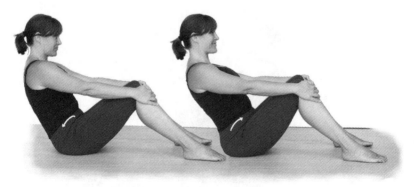

▶ DOORJAMB PULL-UP

• Stand in a doorway and grasp the side of the doorway around shoulder height (as you practice you should vary the height at which you place your arm).

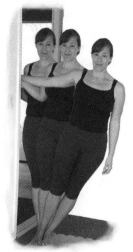 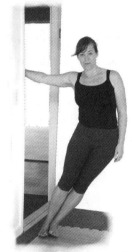

how to do this exercise   *how **not** to do this exercise*

• Keeping your body vertical, your feet together and close to the wall, and your elbow pointing down to the floor (and not behind you), lower your body away from the doorway, and then pull yourself back up. (If you have a tendency to over-extend your elbow, make sure you don't quite straighten all the way.)
• To make the motion less difficult, move your feet away from the wall and start there, moving your feet toward the wall as you get stronger.
• Your core muscles are the ones working to keep your body straight, so the less straight your body, the less core work you'll be doing.

▶ WALL CRESCENT

• Stand against a wall, and get yourself lined up so that, while your feet remain a few inches from the wall, your butt, ribcage, and the back of your head are on the wall.

• Reach your arms over your head until your hands touch the wall above.

• **It's more important for you to keep the legs straight, pelvis neutral, and ribs down than it is for you to touch the wall with your head and hands.** The more you do this, the closer you'll be.

• Now do a side bend, **without any twisting or thrusting,** using the wall as a guide to tell you when you have lost your alignment points.

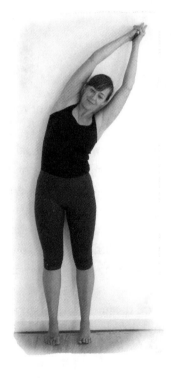

INNER THIGHS

▸ KNEE OUT TO THE SIDE

• Lying face down with your belly on the floor, slide your right knee along the floor until it's out to your side, keeping your right leg bent.

• If your hips are very stiff you might find that you can barely move the thigh without moving the pelvis. **In this case, turn your pelvis so that it "faces" the knee**, and see if you can get it higher.

• Once the knee is closer to your head, turn the pelvis back to the floor, increasing the stretch.

• Hang out in the most comfortable place between knee up to the side and pelvis flat on the ground.

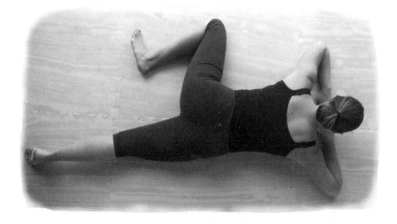

• Repeat on the other side, working up to a few times back and forth, holding each side about a minute.

▶ LEG OUT TO THE SIDE

• Start face down on the floor.

• Following the same instructions as for Knee Out to the Side but with a straight leg, scoot your leg up toward your head, sliding it up along the floor.

• Bring it up as high as you can without lifting one side of the pelvis away from the floor or hiking one hip up toward your ribcage. Try to keep the right and left sides of your waist the same length.

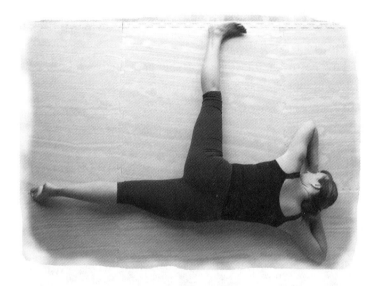

• As you advance, try to externally rotate the stretching leg by rolling your thighbone so the toes on that foot point more toward the ceiling and less toward the floor.

• Rest your head and neck on your hands, hanging out here or in some modified position that allows you to relax.

▶ SUPINE SOLES TOGETHER

• Lying on your back, bolstering the ribs as necessary, bend your knees until the soles of your feet are touching, then drop your knees out to sides.

• **If this is too much of a stretch for your groin, place pillows under each knee to support you in this position.** Lower the support bolsters as the position becomes more comfortable.

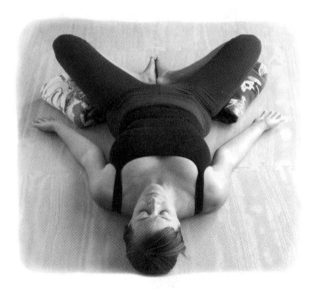

▸ SUPINE STACKED LEGS

- From the position of the last exercise, cross your ankles to place one ankle on top of the opposite shin.
- Let both knees drop toward the floor, **bolstering your knees as necessary**.

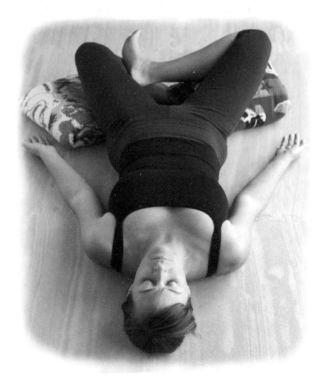

▶ WIDE SQUAT WITH SIT-BACK

- Starting on your hands and knees (don't forget to mind your ribs), widen your knees so they're wider than your pelvis.
- Sit back toward your feet without tucking your pelvis.

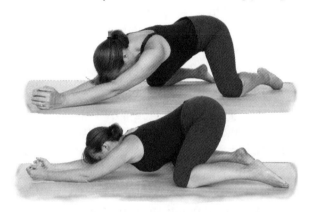

- If you need to, **reduce the load by doing this on a bed or other soft or squishy surface, or place one pillow or blanket behind your knees (so they aren't forced into flexion), and one under your ankles** so that gravity doesn't force you beyond your current ranges of motion.

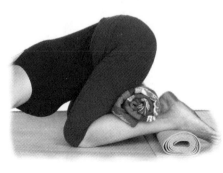

- Once you're as far back as your pelvis can go without tucking, shift your pelvis from side to side, gently, to see if there's any tension deep in the hips.
- You can also do this exercise at different knee-widths; each width provides a different load!

FRONT OF THE THIGH

▸ KNEECAP RELEASE

• Stand with your legs vertical (as on page 66) and let your kneecaps down by relaxing the quadriceps muscles.

• If this is too difficult, get a wall behind you and then let your weight be fully supported by resting your butt against it. If the quads aren't relaxing it's usually because you're still ever-so-slightly bending your knees.

• If the kneecaps are still not dropping, sit on the front edge of a chair and, keeping your heels on the ground, stretch your legs out in front of you. Let the legs fully straighten. See if you can relax your quads in this position.

• Once you've mastered the quad release, it should be added to your other leg-alignment points (feet straight, ankles ASIS width, neutral knee pits)—which isn't easy! You might find that you're tensing your quads to rotate your thigh; ideally this rotation should come from the deeper hip rotators and not require quad use.

▸ ILIACUS RELEASE

- Lie on your back (bolstering your ribs!) with your knees bent.
- Prop the inferior (closer to your legs) half of the pelvis up on a bolster, yoga block, or stack of towels, making sure to leave space under your waistband.
- Like a teeter-totter, your pelvis should tip toward your head, lowering your waistband toward the floor.
- Don't work to rotate the pelvis; this defeats the point of "release." Just allow gravity to create this motion for you.
- Hang out here as long as you like, knowing that even if your pelvis doesn't budge, gravity is still creating the forces necessary to signal "lengthen!" to these muscles.

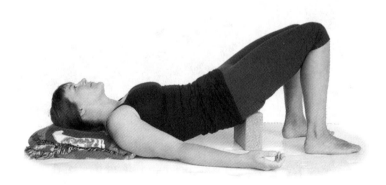

▸ PSOAS RELEASE

• Start by sitting on the floor with legs extended. Relax the muscles of the thighs until the hamstrings (muscles on the back of the thigh) rest on the ground. You might need to untuck your pelvis for this to happen.

• Once your thighs are down, start to recline, stopping just before the hamstrings lift away from the ground. At this angle, bolster your head and shoulders, leaving space for the ribs to lower to the floor.

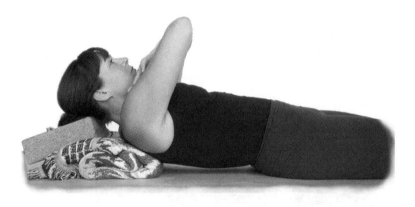

• Once you have bolstered your head and shoulders, start relaxing the ribs to the floor. As with all the other "releasing" exercises, the point is not to get your ribcage to the floor by flexing your muscles, but to realize just how much you're tensing muscles and moving your own skeleton subconsciously.

• As you relax your psoas, your ribs will be able to move closer to the floor, so continuously adjusting the height or position of the bolster will be necessary as you improve.

▸ RECTUS FEMORIS QUAD STRETCH

• Starting on your belly, place a bolster—a rolled-up sleeping bag works great for this—under the front of your pelvis (put your ASIS, a.k.a. "hipbones," higher up on the roll) and let your pubic bone fall toward the floor. This will tilt your pelvis into place, making this next part of the exercise extremely effective.

• To see how much tension is in this one quad, bend your knee, bringing your ankle to your hand, if you can reach it, without letting your pubic bone change position.

• You might find that your foot won't even reach your hand, so to stretch this one muscle, you might need a strap (or a belt or tie) to loop around your ankle so you can reach it with ease.

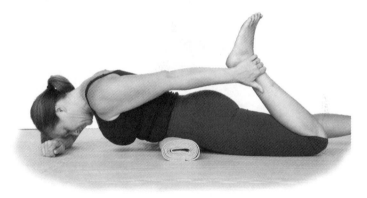

• Grab the lowest part of the shin and not the foot or toes. This will keep you from displacing the load to hyper-lax ankle ligaments instead of the rectus femoris.

▸ THE LUNGE MAKEOVER

• Start by sitting up on your knees, preferably on something soft, like carpet or a yoga mat.
• Step forward with your right leg and shift your weight forward to your front foot, lowering your pelvis toward the floor.
• Repeat other leg.

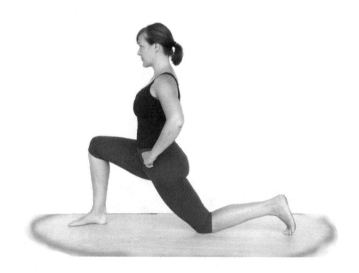

- This time, line up your pelvis so that it is in neutral—keep the ASIS and pubic symphysis on a vertical plane.
- Step forward with your right foot, and shift your weight forward toward the front foot as far as you can without your pelvis tilting.

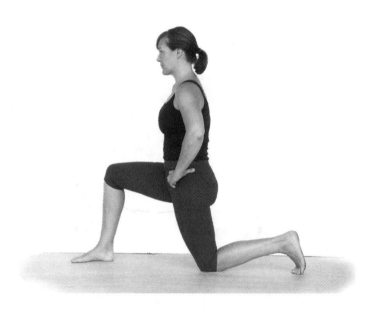

- If you need to, scoot your front foot forward, until you feel your back leg can't extend any farther. Repeat other side.

▸ HIP SLIDE AND GLIDE

• Stand in front of a chair with your feet a little wider than shoulder-width apart and bend forward, resting your hands on the seat.

• Relax the spine down toward the floor, without bending the arms.

• After you've relaxed the spine, back your hips up until they are behind your heels.

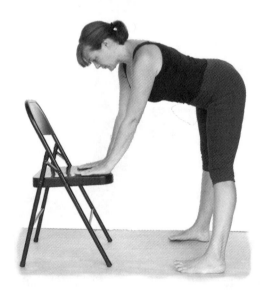

• If your hamstrings are super tight and you find that, even after you relax your spine, your back is rounding up like a cat's, build up the height of the seat with blankets or books until your arms are holding your weight and your spine is relaxed and no longer rounded.

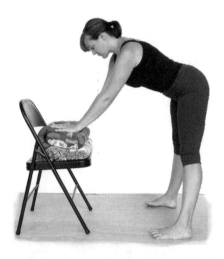

• Shift your pelvis toward the right foot and then toward the left.
• There are two ways to make this more challenging. The first is to rotate your thighs into neutral (as shown on page 68); this will bring your whole leg into a better alignment to load muscles that are affecting how your thigh and pelvis relate to each other when you're walking.
• A second way is to do the Slide and Glide with your butt against a wall to stop you from "cheating" on this exercise.

ABDOMINAL EXERCISES

▸ ROLL OVER, ROLL BACK

• Lie on your back with your legs straight and your arms stretched out over your head.

• Without lifting your head, arms, or legs, initiate a roll to your left and onto your stomach, and then once more in the same direction, so that you end up on your back. Eventually your arms, legs, and head will move, but this exercise is to try to get you to initiate the work from the core muscles—just as you did it when you were a baby.

• Then repeat rolling to the opposite direction.

• Repeat this ten times.

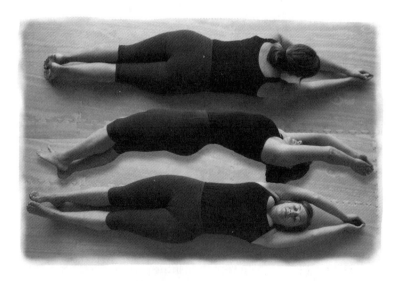

▸ THE ROCKING CHAIR

- Start by lying on your back, with your knees in toward your chest.
- Wrap your arms underneath your shins so that you're holding your thighs close to your body, and then grab each arm's wrist or elbow to keep your legs in place.
- Lift your head and shoulders off the ground, making your body the shape of a rocking chair.
- **Without straining**, rock your body back and forth between the bottom of your ribs and just below your waistband. Do not go any higher or lower than these markers.
- If your floor is especially hard, fold a towel a couple of times to create a softer surface for this area of your spine.
- If you're unable to move at all—if that area of the body won't curve and just stays a flat line—go back and work on the Click-Clack (on page 99) for a few more weeks, then check back to see if this one is getting any easier for you!

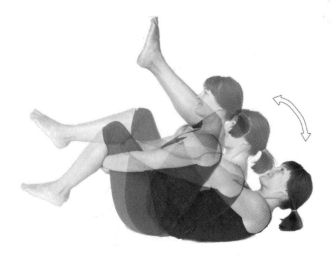

▶ ROCKING CHAIR 360

• Once you've mastered a core-driven rocking chair, start turning yourself around in small increments with every rock until you've spun yourself around 360 degrees.

• Do the same thing in the opposite direction.

• If you notice yourself straining—grunting and gasping and throwing your body forward and back—**you're not ready for this exercise yet**.

• You should be able to breathe easily throughout—a sign that you're not messing with your pressures (and straining your linea alba and/or pelvic floor) while doing this exercise.

SIT BETTER

▸ SIT NEAR THE FRONT OF YOUR CHAIR

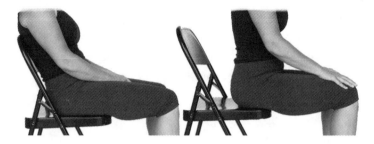

• Scoot your body toward the front of the chair so you are unable to use the spinal support.
• To help you untuck your pelvis, sit right at the front edge of your chair.

▸ UNTUCK YOUR PELVIS

• As you sit on the edge of your chair, roll your pelvis forward as though it's a bowl of soup you're trying to pour out the front, until your ASIS and pubic symphysis are in vertical alignment (a.k.a. "neutral pelvis").

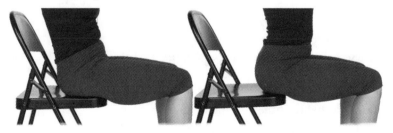

• To make this pelvic motion bigger (i.e., easier to feel), sit on a rolled towel.

▸ DE-HUMP YOUR UPPER BACK

• Keeping your ribs down, work to bring your head and eyes level to the horizon without lifting your chin or moving your ribcage.

• To do this you need to move the vertebrae in the upper back.

• Think of sliding the back of your head to the wall behind you, while lifting the crown of your head up to the ceiling.

SIT DIFFERENTLY

• Sit in many different configurations all day: sit cross-legged on a chair; sit on a bolster or pillow and spread your legs in a wide V; sit directly on the floor; sit on your knees.

• It's okay if you're not able to stay in any one position for long or if you need to add pillows under your hips to make this new way of sitting comfortable. It only matters that you change something about the geometry in your hips.

• Drop your ribs.

SIT LESS

▸ IDEAS TO REDUCE SITTING TIME

• Look for times you can reduce the amount of unnecessary (i.e., non-work) time you spend in a chair.

• Consider eating some meals standing at the counter.

• Lie on the floor or do stretches while you watch TV at night.

• Kneel while you fold laundry instead of sitting on the bed.

- If you take public transit, consider standing for at least some of the journey.
- Walk instead of driving, or drive partway, and walk the rest.

▶ STANDING (DYNAMIC) WORKSTATION

- Try standing up to work for 10 percent of your computer time at first—fifty minutes of an eight-hour day.
- This doesn't have to be all at once—in fact, it will be more beneficial to spread those fifty minutes out over the rest of your work time, changing between standing and sitting fairly frequently.

▶ WALKING

- Increase your mileage gradually and try to eventually walk three to five miles most days, with semi-regular longer walks of eight to ten miles.
- You don't have to do all your walking at once; it's just as beneficial to your core muscles, if not more, to spread it out over the day, breaking up long bouts of stillness.
- Try to blend errands and walking to get a ten- or fifteen-minute walk in here or there.
- Try taking work phone calls and meetings outside for a stroll.

▸ HANGING

- To begin, find a bar or branch that allows you to keep your feet on the ground.
- Holding on with both arms, slowly bend your knees, dropping the weight of your body away from your hands.
- **If your elbows straighten beyond 180°, put a small bend in them and work to maintain it. This will protect the ligaments in your elbows.**

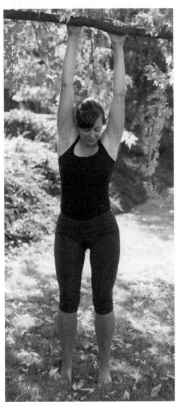

- Once you can stabilize your elbows, find a bar that allows you to hang with your feet off the ground.
- **Check your shoulder blades; are they up at your ears? See if you can bring them down toward your waistband, and see if you can keep your ribs down.**
- When you're hanging with your shoulders and ribs down and you're breathing, you should feel the muscles in your midsection working.

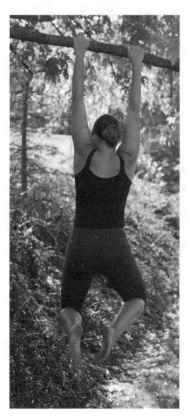

▸ SWINGING

- Once you've mastered the hang, see if you can get your body swinging forward and back.
- Try to work up to ten swings.
- **If you're not able to keep your elbows from over-extending and your shoulders down, then back up a step and practice the static hang more often.**

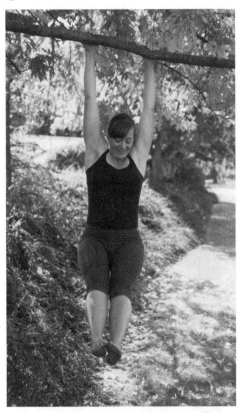

• Another type of swinging, which will better prepare you for one-armed hanging and swinging, is a side-to-side swing.
• Use your waist muscles to get your legs swinging right to left, like a pendulum. Just as in the other hangs and swings, keep the shoulders and the ribs down to better utilize the muscles in your trunk.

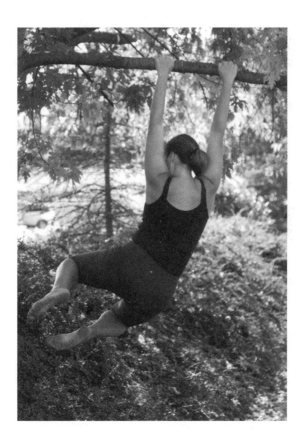

▶ THE MONKEY BARS

- Begin hanging and then swinging from one arm, increasing the strength in both arms.
- **Only progress as your body indicates better strength through better ability to stabilize your elbows.**
- Eventually, go across the monkey bars daily.

▶ CARRYING

- Fix your base. The base of carrying is everything your arms attach to. **Line up your feet and knees, stack your pelvis, drop your ribs, and then assume the load.**
- Constantly shift how you carry. If you're carrying a baby, for example, carry a while on your right and a while on your left side. A while on your back, and a while on your front. The same goes for carrying a backpack or purse. Switch arms, test out your new grip strength and your core in a unique way.
- Carry often. Ditch the stroller and carry your kid in arms, even if it's only for a short period of time. Walk to the grocery store and carry that gallon of milk in your hands instead of in a bag. Stack your own wood in the winter.

▶ GET DOWN, GET UP

- Go sit on the floor.
- Get back up again.
- Go sit on the floor in a different way.
- Get back up again.
- Repeat until you've sat down and gotten up ten times.

▸ **THE SIT AND SHIFT**

• Start sitting with your legs tucked underneath you, with your knees bent and your feet under your bottom.

• Lower your right hip to the right, until it is resting on the ground.

• **If your waist is very tight, bolster this exercise by placing a folded bath towel just to the right and left side of your hips, in which case you only have to lower your right hip to the height of the towel.**

• Sit here for a moment, and then, using the muscles in your waist, lower body, and a little momentum, shift your hips to the left.

• Try to keep your torso upright and your ribs down as you shift from side to side.

• You don't need to do this quickly; rather you're seeing how well you can change the position of your body utilizing the muscles of the waist.

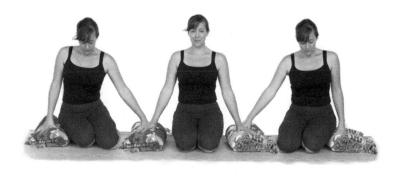

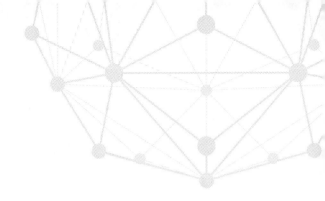

APPENDICES

APPENDIX 1: RECOMMENDED BOOKS AND PRODUCTS

- My favorite layperson anatomy book is *Clinical Anatomy Made Ridiculously Simple,* by Stephen Goldberg, M.D., and Hugue Ouellette, M.D.

- The Squatty Potty is available at squattypotty.com.

Two excellent approaches for self-myofascial release:

- *The Roll Model: A Step-by-Step Guide to Erase Pain, Improve Mobility, and Live Better in Your Body,* by Jill Miller. Jill created Yoga Tune Up® Therapy Balls (they come in many different sizes and you can also find great instructional DVDs for using these at yogatuneup.com).

- *The MELT Method: A Breakthrough Self-Treatment System to Eliminate Chronic Pain, Erase the Signs of Aging, and Feel Fantastic in Just 10 Minutes a Day!,* by Sue Hitzmann. You can find MELT Method products at meltmethod.com.

APPENDIX 2: DIET

I'll start by listing all the folks who contributed tips for the diet section on page 28. I'm grateful to each of them for sharing a bit of their knowledge here, and I recommend you look up any and all of them, as they all have helpful resources available.

- Liz Wolfe is the author of *Eat The Yolks*. Her website, realfoodliz.com, is an amazing learning portal, and she's the co-host of one of my favorite podcasts, Balanced Bites.

- Diane Sanfilippo is the author of NYT bestsellers *The 21-Day Sugar Detox* and *Practical Paleo*. Her excellent website is balancedbites.com and she is—you guessed it—the other co-host of the Balanced Bites podcast.

- Roland Denzel and Galina Denzel are the authors of *The Real Food Reset* and other fantastic books. Their website is EatWellMoveWell.com, and their Eat Well, Move Well articles, podcast, videos, and coaching help clients find true health.

- Amanda Love, The Barefoot Cook, is "an Inspirational Chef-tivist + Dharma teacher for your diet." Her website is thebarefootcook.com, and she offers online and in-person sessions to help people revolutionize how they eat. One of her products is the Nourishing Cleanse, a bone broth–based detox program. Her broth recipe is on page 208.

- Carmina McGee, MS, RDN, is an Integrative Wellness Coach and Nutritionist. At her website, carminamcgee.com, you can see the great coaching and counseling services she offers, and keep up with her blog about all things health and food.

Chicken Bone Broth
by Amanda Love, thebarefootcook.com

Many people think broth and stock are the same thing, but there is, in fact, a difference. Chicken stock is made by simmering the whole chicken, including the skin, bones, and meat. Bone broth is made by simmering just bones and water. It is optional to add veggies and herbs to either bone broth or meat stock.

Making Chicken Bone Broth

Save bones from making chicken meat stock, from roasted chickens, raw chicken backs, or any other bones (that you have ideally roasted prior to making broth). Once you have several carcasses or about 3–5 pounds of bones, you are good to go and can make a strong broth. If you can find chicken feet, this will enhance your broth. Add about 3–5 chicken feet in the pot. This will help add extra gelatin. If you have access to chicken heads, even better. Add a few heads as well.

Ingredients
- 3–5 pounds chicken bones including carcasses, backs, feet, heads—organic or pasture raised
- 2 tablespoons raw apple cider vinegar
- 1 tablespoon good salt
- 4 quarts filtered water (16 cups or 1 gallon)

Optional

Do not add these until the last 2–3 hours of making the broth.
- 1 medium yellow onion, quartered
- 2–4 carrots, halved

- 3–4 celery stalks, halved
- 5 sprigs parsley
- Bouquet garni (fresh bay leaf, fresh sage, rosemary, and thyme. Tie herbs to a carrot or celery stalk with cooking twine for easy removal or place in a little muslin sack.)

Instructions

1. Place 2–3 chicken carcasses or about 3–5 pounds of bones in a stock pot as well as feet and heads if you can find them.
2. Cover with a gallon of water.
3. Add 2 tablespoons raw apple cider vinegar.
4. Add 1 tablespoon good salt.
5. Bring to a low simmer.
6. If you want to add any veggies and/or herbs for added flavor and nutrition, wait to do so until the last 2–3 hours of cooking or else your broth will have an "off" flavor. (Adding herbs and veggies is optional.)
7. Simmer on low heat so broth is just barely bubbling for 12–24 hours.
8. Strain and cool. See storage tips from above.

Instructions

Store in pint size large mouth mason jars (a great size for quick thawing) or any kind of glass storage containers. The stock will last about 1 week in the fridge or 3 months in the freezer. The more gelatinous the broth, the longer it will last.

Some research on the benefits of bone broth:

Bannai, M., & Kawai, N. (2011). New therapeutic strategy for amino acid medicine: glycine improves the quality of sleep- *Journal of Pharmacological Sciences 118*, 145–148.

Brind, J., Malloy, V., Augie, I., Caliendo, N., Vogelman, J. H., Zimmerman, J. A., Orentreich, N. (2011). Dietary glycine supplementation mimics lifespan extension by dietary methionine restriction in Fisher 344 rats. *The FASEB Journal, 25, 528.2.*

Clark, K. L., Sebastianelli, W., Flechsenhar, K.R., et al. (2008). 24-Week study on the use of collagen hydrolysate as a dietary supplement in athletes with activity-related joint pain. *Curr Med Res Opin. May;24*(5), 1485-96.

Vieira, C. P., Oliveira, L. P. D., Guerra, F. D. R., Almeida, M. D. S. D., Marcondes, M. C. C. G. and Pimentel, E. R. (2015). Glycine Improves Biochemical and Biomechanical Properties Following Inflammation of the Achilles Tendon. *Anat Rec, 298*, 538–545.

REFERENCES AND
FURTHER READING

Akram, J., & Matzen, S. H. (2014). Rectus abdominis diastasis. *Journal of Plastic Surgery and Hand Surgery, 48*(3), 163-169.

Axer, H., von Keyserlingk, D. G., & Prescher, A. (2001). Collagen Fibers in Linea Alba and Rectus Sheaths: I. General Scheme and Morphological Aspects. *Journal of Surgical Research, 96*(1), 127-134.

Axer, H., von Keyserlingk, D. G., & Prescher, A. (2001). Collagen fibers in linea alba and rectus sheaths. *Journal of Surgical Research, 96*(2), 239-245.

Barbosa, S., de Sa, R. A., & Coca Velarde, L. G. (2013). Diastasis of rectus abdominis in the immediate puerperium: correlation between imaging diagnosis and clinical examination. *Archives of Gynecology and Obstetrics, 288*(2), 299-303.

Beer, G. M., Schuster, A., Seifert, B., Manestar, M., Mihic-Probst, D., & Weber, S. A. (2009). The normal width of the linea alba in nulliparous women. *Clinical Anatomy, 22*(6), 706-711.

Bellido Luque, J., Bellido Luque, A., Valdivia, J., Suarez Grau, J. M., Gomez Menchero, J., Garcia Moreno, J., & Guadalajara Jurado, J. (2014). Totally endoscopic surgery on diastasis recti associated with midline hernias. The advantages of a minimally invasive approach. Prospective cohort study. *Hernia 19*(3), 493-501.

Benjamin, D. R., van de Water, A. T. M., & Peiris, C. L. (2014). Effects of exercise on diastasis of the rectus abdominis muscle in the antenatal and postnatal periods: a systematic review. *Physiotherapy, 100*(1), 1-8.

Blanchard, P. D. (2005). Diastasis recti abdominis in HIV-infected men with lipodystrophy. *HIV Medicine, 6*(1), 54-56.

Boissonnault, J. S., & Blaschak, M. J. (1988). Incidence of diastasis recti abdominis during the childbearing year. *Physical Therapy, 68*(7), 1082-1086.

Brauman, D. (2008). Diastasis recti: clinical anatomy. *Plastic and Reconstructive Surgery, 122*(5), 1564-1569.

Bugenstein, R. H., & Phibbs, C. M., Jr. (1975). Abdominal pain in children caused by linea alba hernias. *Pediatrics, 56*(6), 1073-1074.

Chiarello, C. M., Falzone, L. A., McCaslin, K. E., Patel, M. N., & Ulery, K. R. (2005). The Effects of an Exercise Program on Diastasis Recti Abdominis in Pregnant Women. *Journal of Women's Health Physical Therapy, 29*(1), 11-16. Retrieved from: journals.lww.com/jwhpt/Fulltext/2005/29010/The_Effects_of_an_Exercise_Program_on_Diastasis.3.aspx

Chiarello, C. M., & McAuley, J. A. (2013). Concurrent validity of calipers and ultrasound imaging to measure interrecti distance. *Journal of Orthopaedic and Sports Physical Therapy, 43*(7), 495-503.

Cholewicki, J., Juluru, K., & McGill, S. M. (1999). Intra-abdominal pressure mechanism for stabilizing the lumbar spine. *Journal of Biomechanics, 32*(1), 13-17.

Chun, R., Baghirzada, L., Tiruta, C., & Kirkpatrick, A. W. (2012). Measurement of intra-abdominal pressure in term pregnancy: a pilot study. *International Journal of Obstetric Anesthesia, 21*(2), 135-139.

Cobb, W. S., Burns, J. M., Kercher, K. W., Matthews, B. D., James Norton, H., & Todd Heniford, B. (2005). Normal Intraabdominal Pressure in Healthy Adults. *Journal of Surgical Research, 129*(2), 231-235.

Cohen, M. M., Jr. (2005). Beckwith-Wiedemann syndrome: historical, clinicopathological, and etiopathogenetic perspectives. *Pediatric and Developmental Pathology, 8*(3), 287-304.

Coldron, Y., Stokes, M. J., Newham, D. J., & Cook, K. (2008). Postpartum characteristics of rectus abdominis on ultrasound imaging. *Manual Therapy, 13*(2), 112-121.

Davis, B. B. (1895). V. Hernia in the Linea Alba. *Annals of Surgery, 21*(4), 464-467.

Digilio, M. C., Capolino, R., & Dallapiccola, B. (2008). Autosomal dominant transmission of nonsyndromic diastasis recti and weakness of the linea alba. *American Journal of Medical Genetics, A, 146a*(2), 254-256.

Essendrop, M., Andersen, T. B., & Schibye, B. (2002). Increase in spinal stability obtained at levels of intra-abdominal pressure and back muscle activity realistic to work situations. *Applied Ergonomics, 33*(5), 471-476.

Fachinelli, A., Trindade, M. R., & Fachinelli, F. A. (2011). Elastic fibers in the anterior abdominal wall. *Hernia, 15*(4), 409-415.

Förstemann, T., Trzewik, J., Holste, J., Batke, B., Konerding, M. A., Wolloscheck, T., & Hartung, C. (2011). Forces and deformations of the abdominal wall—A mechanical and geometrical approach to the linea alba. *Journal of Biomechanics, 44*(4), 600-606.

Gräβel, D., Prescher, A., Fitzek, S., Keyserlingk, D. G. v., & Axer, H. (2005). Anisotropy of human linea alba: A biomechanical study. *Journal of Surgical Research, 124*(1), 118-125.

Hernandez-Gascon, B., Mena, A., Pena, E., Pascual, G., Bellon, J. M., & Calvo, B. (2013). Understanding the passive mechanical behavior of the human abdominal wall. *Annals of Biomedical Engineering, 41*(2), 433-444.

Hickey, F., Finch, J. G., & Khanna, A. (2011). A systematic review on the outcomes of correction of diastasis of the recti. *Hernia, 15*(6), 607-614.

Hodges, P. W., Eriksson, A. E. M., Shirley, D., & Gandevia, S. C. (2005). Intra-abdominal pressure increases stiffness of the lumbar spine. *Journal of Biomechanics, 38*(9), 1873-1880.

Hodges, P. W., & Gandevia, S. C. (2000). Changes in intra-abdominal pressure during postural and respiratory activation of the human diaphragm. *Journal of Applied Physiology (1985), 89*(3), 967-976.

Hollinsky, C., & Sandberg, S. (2007). Measurement of the tensile strength of the ventral abdominal wall in comparison with scar tissue. *Clinical Biomechanics, 22*(1), 88-92.

Hsia, M., & Jones, S. (2000). Natural resolution of rectus abdominis diastasis. Two single case studies. *Australian Journal of Physiotherapy, 46*(4), 301-307.

Konerding, M. A., Bohn, M., Wolloscheck, T., Batke, B., Holste, J.-L., Wohlert, S.... Hartung, C. (2011). Maximum forces acting on the abdominal wall: Experimental validation of a theoretical modeling in a human cadaver study. *Medical Engineering & Physics, 33*(6), 789-792.

Korenkov, M., Beckers, A., Koebke, J., Lefering, R., Tiling, T., & Troidl, H. (2001). Biomechanical and morphological types of the linea alba and its possible role in the pathogenesis of midline incisional hernia. *European Journal of Surgery, 167*(12), 909-914.

Kulhanek, J., & Mestak, O. (2013). Treatment of umbilical hernia and recti muscles diastasis without a periumbilical incision. *Hernia, 17*(4), 527-530.

Lehnert, B., Wadouh, F. (1992). High coincidence of inguinal hernias and abdominal aortic aneurysms. *Annals of Vascular Surgery, 6*, 134–7.

Leong, D. P., Teo, K. K., Rangarajan, S., Lopez-Jaramillo, P., Avezum, A., Orlandini, A., Seron, P., Ahmed, S. H., Rosengren, A., Kelishadi, R., Rahman, O., Swaminathan, S., Iqbal, R., Gupta, R., Lear, S. A., Oguz, A., Yusoff, K., Zatonska, K., Chifamba, J., Igumbor, E., Mohan, V., Mohan Anjana, R., Gu, H., Li, W., Yusuf, S. (2015). Prognostic value of grip strength: findings from the Prospective Urban Rural Epidemiology (PURE) study. *The Lancet, 386(9990)*, 266–273.

Liaw, L. J., Hsu, M. J., Liao, C. F., Liu, M. F., & Hsu, A. T. (2011). The relationships between inter-recti distance measured by ultrasound imaging and abdominal muscle function in postpartum women: a 6-month follow-up study. *Journal of Orthopaedic and Sports Physical Therapy, 41*(6), 435-443.

Lovering, R. M. & Anderson, L. D. (2008) Architecture and fiber type of the pyramidalis muscle. *Anatomical Scientific International, 83*(4), 294-7.

McPhail, I. (2008). Abdominal aortic aneurysm and diastasis recti. *Angiology, 59*(6), 736-739.

Mendes Dde, A., Nahas, F. X., Veiga, D. F., Mendes, F. V., Figueiras, R. G., Gomes, H. C.... Ferreira, L. M. (2007). Ultrasonography for measuring rectus abdominis muscles diastasis. *Acta Cirurgica Brasileira, 22*(3), 182-186.

Moesbergen, T., Law, A., Roake, J., & Lewis, D. R. (2009). Diastasis recti and abdominal aortic aneurysm. *Vascular, 17*(6), 325-329.

Mota, P., Pascoal, A. G., Sancho, F., & Bo, K. (2012). Test-retest and intrarater reliability of 2-dimensional ultrasound measurements of distance between rectus abdominis in women. *Journal of Orthopaedic and Sports Physical Therapy, 42*(11), 940-946.

Mota, P., Pascoal, A. G., Sancho, F., Carita, A. I., & Bø, K. (2013). Reliability of the inter-rectus distance measured by palpation. Comparison of palpation and ultrasound measurements. *Manual Therapy, 18*(4), 294-298.

Mota, P. G., Pascoal, A. G., Carita, A. I., & Bo, K. (2015). Prevalence and risk factors of diastasis recti abdominis from late pregnancy to 6 months postpartum, and relationship with lumbo-pelvic pain. *Manual Therapy, 20*(1), 200-205.

Nahas, F. X. (1996). Studies on the endoscopic correction of diastasis recti. *Operative Techniques in Plastic and Reconstructive Surgery, 3*(1), 58-61.

Nahas, F. X., Augusto, S. M., & Ghelfond, C. (1997). Should diastasis recti be corrected? *Aesthetic Plastic Surgery, 21*(4), 285-289.

Naraynsingh, V., Maharaj, R., Dan, D., & Hariharan, S. (2012). Strong linea alba: Myth or reality? *Medical Hypotheses, 78*(2), 291-292. doi:http://dx.doi.org/10.1016/j.mehy.2011.11.004

Parker, M. A., Millar, L. A., & Dugan, S. A. (2009). Diastasis Rectus Abdominis and Lumbo-Pelvic Pain and Dysfunction—Are They Related? *Journal of Women's Health Physical Therapy, 33*(2), 15-22.

Pascoal, A. G., Dionisio, S., Cordeiro, F., & Mota, P. (2014). Inter-rectus distance in postpartum women can be reduced by isometric contraction of the abdominal muscles: a preliminary case-control study. *Physiotherapy, 100*(4), 344-348.

Ranney, B. (1990). Diastasis recti and umbilical hernia causes, recognition and repair. *South Dakota Journal of Medicine, 43*(10), 5-8.

Rath, A. M., Attali, P., Dumas, J. L., Goldlust, D., Zhang, J., & Chevrel, J. P. (1996). The abdominal linea alba: an anatomo-radio-logic and biomechanical study. *Surgical and Radiologic Anatomy, 18*(4), 281-288.

Spitznagle, T. M., Leong, F. C., & Van Dillen, L. R. (2007). Prev-alence of diastasis recti abdominis in a urogynecological patient population. *International Urogynecology Journal, 18*(3), 321-328.

Stokes, I. A., Gardner-Morse, M. G., & Henry, S. M. (2010). Intra-abdominal pressure and abdominal wall muscular func-tion: Spinal unloading mechanism. *Clinical Biomechanics, 25*(9), 859-866.

Tokita, K. (2006). Anatomical significance of the nerve to the pyramidalis muscle: a morphological study. *Anatomical Science International, 81*(4), 210-24.

Verissimo, P., Nahas, F. X., Barbosa, M. V., de Carvalho Gomes, H. F., & Ferreira, L. M. (2014). Is it possible to repair diastasis recti and shorten the aponeurosis at the same time? *Aesthetic Plastic Surgery, 38*(2), 379-386.

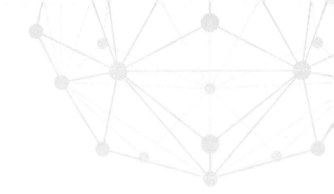

INDEX

diaphragam, 38, 40, 74-77, 91, 165
diet,
    food, 28-30, 48-49, 51, 60, 207, 210
    movement, 39, 48-49, 51-54, 60
digestion, 30, 42, 79
Doorjamb Pull-Up (little move), 102-103, 177
Doorway Walkthrough (exercise), 86-87, 168
driving, 23, 41, 49, 139, 197
Drop Your Ribs (body neutral), 41, 71-74, 155
dynamic workstation (big moves), 140, 197

E
equipment list, 58
exercise/therapy balls, 58, 69, 151- 153, 206

F
fascia, 5, 14, 19, 58, 151, 153, 206
fat, abdominal, 23, 27-31, 34, 36, 39, 53, 75
Feet Pelvis-Width Apart (body neutral), 64
Floor Angels (little move), 84, 166
Floor Crescent (little move), 93-94, 171
floor sitting, 52, 60, 139, 148, 196, 202
furniture, 50, 135, 136, 148

G
gait/gait pattern, 45
gelatin, 30, 208-209
Get Down, Get Up (big move), 148, 202
grip strength, 146, 147, 202

rotation
    of femurs/thighs, 68, 108, 115, 125, 162, 180, 184, 191
    of pelvis, 101, 116, 176, 185
    of ribs, 73
    of shoulders, 86, 88
    of spine, *see* twisting

S
Sanfilippo, Diane, 29, 207
shoes, 6, 22, 28, 43, 45, 47, 50, 62-63, 68, 114, 157
Sit and Shift (big move), 148-150, 203
sit better, 135
sit differently, 138-139
sit less, 139
Sit Near the Front of Your Chair (big move), 136, 195
sitting time, 133-134, 139-140, 196-197
smoking, 59, 61, 126
soda/diet soda, 28
Spinal Twist (little moves)
    bolstered, 96-97, 173
    seated, 94-95, 172
squat/squatting, xiii, 6, 52, 60, 139, 206, (as exercise: 112, 183)
stabilization, 151
    of abdominal muscle attachment sites, 126
    of elbows, 144, 146, 199, 202
    of linea alba, 18
    of ribcage, 90
    of spine, 80
standing workstation, *see* dynamic workstation
stomach, pulling/sucking in, 38, 44, 74-75

U

Untuck Your Pelvis (big move), 137, 195

W

waist, 19, 25, 33, 38, 41, 93-95, 108, 111, 145, 150-153, 171, 180, 201, 203

walking, 2, 51, 52, 60, 61, 64, 67-69, 125, 139, 140-142, 147, 149, 191, 197, 202

walking buddy, 141

Wall Crescent (little move), 103-104, 178

water, 28-30, 49, 208, 209

Weaver, Sigourney 27

Whole Body Barefoot, 69, 225

Wide Squat With Sit-Back (medium move), 112-113, 183

Windmill Stretch (little move), 85, 167

Wolfe, Liz 28-29, 207

Y

Yoga Tune Up®, 58, 152, 206

ABOUT KATY

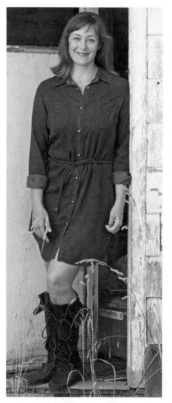

A biomechanist by training and a problem-solver at heart, Katy has the ability to blend a scientific approach with straight talk about sensible solutions and an unwavering sense of humor, earning her legions of followers. Her award-winning blog and podcast, Katy Says, reach hundreds of thousands of people every month, and thousands have taken her live classes. Her books, the bestselling *Move Your DNA* (2014), *Don't Just Sit There* (2015), *Whole Body Barefoot* (2015), *Alignment Matters* (2013), and *Every Woman's Guide to Foot Pain Relief* (2011), have been critically acclaimed and translated worldwide. In between her book-writing efforts, Katy directs and teaches at the Nutritious Movement Center Northwest, travels the globe to teach the Nutritious Movement™ courses in person, and spends as much time outside as possible with her husband and two young children.